Praise for this book

'You don't need to be depressed to benefit from this book. It's full of realistic techniques to help you flourish and reach your potential in life, whatever your emotional starting point. It's easy to do and a guaranteed way to lift your mood at any point in the day.'

Sally Brown, Psychotherapist and Personal Development Coach

'A wonderful set of ideas and techniques that can help reduce depression and build happiness. The techniques are simple, engaging, practical and – most importantly – they're all based on evidence from the latest positive psychology research, so we know they really work.'

Dr Mark Williamson, Director of Action for Happiness

'If I was going to buy one book on positive psychology to treat depression, I'd choose an author who'd been properly trained as a positive psychologist, who knows how to write in an engaging and accessible way, and who understands, first-hand, the challenges of depression. In short, I'd choose Miriam.'

Dr Phil Hammond, GP, BBC broadcaster and author of *Staying Alive: How to Get the Best from the NHS*

'This book was uplifting and offered many helpful tools for a better understanding of the way my brain can help me when I use the power of positive thought. Being mindful takes practise but this book puts us in the driving seat and gives us the understanding needed to methodically change our perceptions of the world. What is so clear is that it's not just our environment or our experiences that make us feel sad or weak ... it's what we think about them.'

Caryn Franklin MBE, Fashion and Identity Commentator, Professor at Kingston School of Art

'This book is a joy. Miriam Akhtar clearly demonstrates that positive psychology is both practical and effective ... in supporting people to recover their wellbeing.'

Amanda Williamson, Director of POW (Positive Opportunities for Wellbeing)

'The first to apply positive psychology solutions to depression, Miriam's book is clear, engaging, enlightening ... and really brings positive psychology to life.'

Dr Ilona Boniwell, Programme Leader, MSc in Applied Positive Psychology, Anglia Ruskin University

'Miriam Akhtar has written a very credible depression treatment manual, based on the principles of positive psychology. I am sure that this book will go on to become one of the few classics in this field … Highly recommended!'

Professor Jerome Carson, Clinical Psychologist

'Miriam Akhtar introduces a major breakthrough in the treatment of depression.'

Dr Chris Johnstone, medical doctor and resilience specialist

'This very readable and thoroughly sensible book will help people to manage their thinking and their lifestyle so that they reduce their current depression and reduce the risk of future distress.'

Professor Neil Frude, Consultant Clinical Psychologist and founder of the Books on Prescription scheme

Dedicated to all those who have ever been visited by the black dog. You are not alone.

Also by Miriam Akhtar

What is Post-Traumatic Growth?
The Happiness Training Plan audio programme
www.happinesstrainingplan.com

POSITIVE PSYCHOLOGY
for Overcoming Depression

**Self-help Strategies to
Build Strength, Resilience
and Sustainable Happiness**

MIRIAM AKHTAR, MAPP

WATKINS
Sharing Wisdom Since 1893

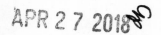
First published 2012.
This revised edition first published in the UK and USA 2018 by
Watkins, an imprint of Watkins Media Limited
19 Cecil Court
London WC2N 4EZ

enquiries@watkinspublishing.com

1 3 5 7 9 10 8 6 4 2

Designed and typeset by Clare Thorpe

Printed and bound in the United Kingdom

A CIP record for this book is available from the British Library

ISBN: 978-1-78678-146-8

www.watkinspublishing.com

Contents

Foreword

Medicine is far too obsessed with what makes us sick, and not nearly interested enough in what keeps us well. Working as a doctor is like camping beside a river. People float downstream and we dive deeper and deeper to pull out those who are sicker and sicker. And we're so busy and exhausted that no one has time to wander upstream and look at what's pushing people in. Depression is one of the biggest challenges facing us and the treatment desperately needs to move upstream. Everyone who's suffered from depression knows that tablets alone aren't the solution. But what is?

You will find the answer in this superb book. Positive psychology focuses on the science of what keeps us mentally healthy and happy. The beauty of this approach, as both a treatment for and preventative of depression, is that it's easy to understand, makes intuitive sense and – most importantly – there's solid scientific evidence to show that it works. It isn't happy-clappy psychobabble but is based on properly researched techniques and mindsets that can keep depression at bay.

In a nutshell, the research shows that if you focus on positive aspects of your life, this can reduce the negative emotions and feelings. I drag myself out of the doldrums with music, books, films, family and walks with the snout of a damp Labrador against my thigh. Modest pleasures, connecting with others and having a sense of meaning and purpose seem to keep me away from the Prozac. It was only when I read this book that I realized a lot of the things I instinctively do to stay positive have been proven to work and yet I rarely discuss them with patients. But I will now.

I've met lots of people with depression over the years, many of whom have been greatly helped by medication, at least in the short term, but all of whom are looking for ways to help themselves. As a family doctor, I have ten minutes (or six by the time the double-buggy is in and out the door) for each consultation and there's never enough time to go into any depth as to what might help my patient be happier and more resilient. This book, however, explores these questions in detail, and with sensitivity, and deserves to become a good friend to anyone who wants to improve their mental health. The question then is whether you can learn the benefits of positive psychology from a book, or whether you have to shell out for a happiness coach or therapist?

My advice is to give this book a go. If I were going to buy one book on positive psychology to treat depression,

I'd choose an author who has been properly trained as a positive psychologist, who knows how to write in an engaging and accessible way, and who understands, first-hand, the challenges of depression. In short, I'd choose Miriam. And if she went into every classroom in the country and taught children how to be resilient, happy and humane, I'd be pulling far fewer bodies out of the river later in life.

Dr Phil Hammond
Doctor, journalist, broadcaster and comedian
www.drphilhammond.com

Appreciation

I'd like to express my gratitude to all those who have contributed to the book. To the academics whose work inspires the positive approach to depression and to my fellow practitioners and colleagues in the world of positive psychology, in particular, for this edition Prof Bob Emmons, Dr Chris Johnstone, Dr Tayyab Rashid, Dr Katie Hanson, Prof Helena Marujo, Prof Luis Miguel Neto and Prof Neil Frude.

I don't find writing easy – it's more meaning than pleasure, even though one of my top strengths is Writer, apparently! So I'd like to thank the friends who keep me going – Ashley Akin-Smith, Ann-Marie Evans, Ginette Ruthven, Chris Samsa, Molly Thompson, Maggie Jeffrey, Jen Gash, Shona Harris and Miranda Steed.

Thank you also to Kelly Thompson and all the other lovely people at Watkins Media.

And to Archie Fischer and Oskar Ruthven. Such a pleasure to see what fine young men you are becoming.

Preface

Since the first edition of this book was published in 2012 there has been a welcome shift in how we treat depression. I remember being keen to broaden knowledge of alternatives to what I saw as a virtual duopoly – either anti-depressant pills or therapy. My own experience of taking anti-depressants, when I was at my most vulnerable – I'd had episodes of depression following a series of losses and the realization that my job no longer suited me – had been a let-down with no real improvement and nasty side-effects. Going into therapy had been surprisingly counterproductive. I knew what was wrong in my life and understood why I was depressed, but picking at my wounds in counselling sessions left me feeling like I was drowning in unhappiness rather than moving on from it. The idea behind the book was to share some practical, evidence-based tools from positive psychology that research has shown can help raise and recover well-being.

Positive psychology has two major advantages to offer anyone at risk of or suffering from depression. Its approach is largely focused on practices that increase well-being, which will be a relief for anyone who prefers doing something that will make them feel better rather than endlessly probing the source of their distress. And the practices work as natural anti-depressants, which will appeal to those who prefer to avoid drug treatment.

I first came across positive psychology as a BBC radio producer making a programme about the science of happiness. This was before it had developed into a new field in psychology. I was intrigued to discover that researchers were applying the same scientific method to investigate the characteristics of well-being as had been applied to studying mental disorders and illness. It made a lot of sense to me. Here, at last, was evidence concerning what it takes to grow your happiness and well-being. My interest wasn't only professional. My deeper motivation was to find a solution to my own multiple episodes of depression. The childhood trauma of my father's sudden death had left me vulnerable in adulthood to depression, which seemed to accompany major transitions and periods of uncertainty in my life. I wondered what the science of happiness could offer someone like me?

I read up on the research and tried out the techniques in this book and was relieved to find that they worked. The effect was gradual, like a dimmer switch slowly turning on the light, but no less substantial for it. Since then, apart from feeling down every so often – a natural part of being human – I've not had another episode of depression.

Not only did I find the key to my recovery but I also discovered my new vocation – to put people on the path to happiness. Prof Martin Seligman, the co-founder of positive psychology, established a Masters in Applied Positive Psychology (MAPP) at the University of Pennsylvania with a goal to train the world's first positive psychologists: *'Individuals whose practice will make the world a happier place, parallel to the way clinical psychologists have made the world a less unhappy place.'*[1] I graduated from the MAPP course at the University of East London and became one of the first positive psychologists in practice in Europe. I still work as a coach and trainer helping people to feel good, function well and flourish. I also have other roles – as a visiting lecturer training up the next generation of positive psychology practitioners and working with professionals, from clinicians to coaches, to teach them about the science and its tools.

In the early years, positive psychology was best known as 'the science of happiness' and became hugely popular – happiness was the new rich, and the symbol most associated with it was the yellow smiley emoji. There came a backlash and it was labelled as 'happyology', accused of fostering a 'tyranny of the positive'. I felt a pressure to be a cheerleader for happiness when, in reality, I was a positive psychologist with a history of depression. Now the field has broadened and, in particular, is known for its work on resilience, or how to cope positively with adversity. We have entered the era of the 'second wave' in positive psychology, symbolized by the yin and yang, which shows how well-being is a complex interplay of the dynamics between positive and negative, light and shade. This, to me, seems to be a much more compassionate and nuanced approach to the human condition, reflecting how joy and sadness can and do co-exist, that there can be a positive in the negative and a negative in the positive. For long-term well-being we are better off facing up to the dark side of human existence rather than trying to deny it. Indeed, the silver lining is that we can, in fact, grow through adversity, and this went on to be the subject of my next book *What is Post-Traumatic Growth?*[2]

My interest has always been in using scientifically-grounded strategies to help people recover their well-being as this had worked for me. I recognize now that I was operating as a second wave positive psychologist before the term was coined.

The first edition of this book, in 2012, broke new ground in terms of looking at how we treat depression and it has meant a great deal to me to hear from readers who've found it helpful and from health professionals and coaches who use the book with their patients and clients. Many of the practices outlined, such as mindfulness, are now mainstream and familiar to many people. Furthermore, a bibliotherapy study (books as therapy) carried out by Sheffield Hallam University actually provided evidence that this book, alongside Prof Paul Gilbert's CBT-based *Overcoming Depression*, reduces symptoms of depression and improves well-being (when one chapter per week was read for eight weeks).[3] It's great to have confirmation that this approach really does work and of the value of books as evidence-based self-help.

For this second edition I've made a number of changes to reflect how the field has matured and how my own practice as a positive psychologist has developed. I've also included new research, in particular in the field of neuroscience. Although depression is depressingly common, it is a unique experience for every individual who suffers and different tools will work for different people – this is reflected in the range of chapters here.

There's an old Native American legend that sums up very well how positive psychology practices work. In the Tale of Two Wolves an old man is teaching his grandson about life. He explains, 'There is a fight going on inside us all between two wolves. One is evil – he is anger, envy, sorrow and regret. The other is good – he is joy, peace, love, hope, serenity, kindness, compassion and faith.' The grandson thinks for a minute and then asks, 'Which wolf wins?' The grandfather replies simply, 'The one you feed.' Positive psychology works by directing your focus toward increasing well-being – by feeding your good wolf.

This book combines knowledge and tools from my professional practice as a positive psychologist and coach with insights gained from my personal experience of spending half a lifetime trying to escape the 'black dog'. Now it's rare for me to feel low and when I do dip down I bounce back faster. I have developed my capacity for happiness and am insulated against depression. I hope this approach works for you too.

Miriam
www.positivepsychologytraining.co.uk

A Positive Approach to Depression

IF YOU THINK YOU HAVE depression you are not alone. The 21st century is in the grip of an epidemic of depression. Over 300 million people are suffering worldwide, making depression the leading cause of ill health. One in two adults in the developed world will experience an episode in their lifetime and having one incidence of depression raises the risk of future episodes. Depression can strike across the lifespan – no longer a phenomenon that emerges in mid-life, the average age for the first onset of depression has fallen to the early teens.

Our modern culture makes us vulnerable to depression. Western society places a high value on happiness, while at the same time we are experiencing record levels of depression. The problem arises when we come to believe that we should always feel happy. This can make us feel ashamed of our negative emotions.

So, sadness is no longer seen as a feeling you expect to have when things go wrong but is interpreted as a sign of failure; a signal something is wrong with you emotionally. People feel a social pressure to be happy – the paradox is that feeling pressure *not* to be depressed is associated with a higher incidence of depressive symptoms.

How do you know if you have depression?

It is natural to feel sad or down, often in response to a loss, an ending, a disappointment or something going wrong in a major area of life, such as relationships or work. The feelings will generally subside with the passage of time. However, depression is *not* the same as this kind of unhappiness. Depression is a constant experience of feeling hopeless, helpless and worthless, which can persist for weeks, months or years, interfering with daily life; affecting how you feel on the inside and how you live your life on the outside. The world takes on a grey, leaden feel that weighs heavy on the body, turns the mind to bleak thoughts and saps the spirit of all meaning in life. It's like falling into a black hole that sucks the joy out of living and leaves you unable to function normally.

So how do you know if you are experiencing depression? You might have been feeling sad, anxious, overwhelmed or pessimistic for a while. It could be that you've lost interest in the things you used to enjoy. You may be physically exhausted, tearful and lethargic. You might be withdrawing into yourself and minimizing contact with others. You may be in despair, crippled by negative thoughts and unable to see anything positive in the future. Any and all of these are symptoms of depression and you might be able to spot others in the list below. You may not even recognize that you're depressed. It might take someone else to point out that you haven't been your usual self for a while or for a doctor to link the signs and make a diagnosis. The symptoms of depression can be quite complex and vary from one person to the next, but probably the most widely recognized is a persistent low mood and loss of enjoyment. If this has been going on for more than two weeks, is causing you distress and affecting your functioning, then these are signs that a doctor might typically use to diagnose depression.

Psychological symptoms of depression include:

- persistent low mood or sadness
- loss of interest or enjoyment of life
- feeling upset
- feeling numb or empty
- feeling hopeless or helpless
- feeling anxious or worried
- feeling irritable and intolerant of others
- low self-esteem or feeling worthless
- poor concentration
- lack of motivation

→

- excessive or inappropriate guilt
- difficulty in making decisions
- thinking about harming yourself
- recurring thoughts of death
- suicidal thoughts

Physical symptoms include:
- tiredness, exhaustion, lack of energy
- tearfulness
- disturbed sleep patterns
- unexplained aches and pains
- moving or speaking more slowly
- restlessness/agitation
- changes in appetite and weight – gain or loss
- lack of self-care
- digestive problems
- low libido
- changes in the menstrual cycle

Social symptoms include:
- a decline in work performance
- difficulties in home life
- avoiding contact with friends
- engaging in fewer social activities
- neglecting your hobbies and interests
- withdrawing or isolating yourself from others

What causes depression?

Although depression is known as 'the common cold of mental health', the mechanics of it are not always easy to identify. Doctors tend to focus on treating the symptoms rather than the underlying reasons for depression. These underlying factors can vary from physical causes, such as the impact of long-term stress on the immune system, infection, brain injuries and diseases such as dementia, to psychological triggers, such as loneliness, grief, traumatic events and romantic rejection. People often blame themselves, interpreting the fact that they have depression as a personal failure on their part. However, negative self-talk like "*it's all my fault*" and "*if only I wasn't like this*" is more likely to be a sign of depression rather than the root cause.

There are many potential triggers to depression such as adverse life events, relationship difficulties, physical health problems and the impact of chronic stress, but in many cases the exact cause of the depression is unknown. According to *The Upward Spiral*, Alex Korb's book on the neuroscience behind depression, the trigger appears to involve a problem with how the brain's thinking circuit (the prefrontal cortex) and its feeling circuit (the limbic system) are working together. To put it simply, the 'thinking' prefrontal cortex is supposed to help regulate the 'feeling' limbic system but they get out of whack in the way they act and communicate with each other.

Two main schools of thought have evolved about the causes of, and consequently the treatment for, depression. Firstly, the biomedical model explains depression primarily as the result of a chemical imbalance in the brain. Sufferers are thought to have low levels of neurotransmitters that affect the mood and are treated with anti-depressants such as SSRIs (Selective Serotonin Reuptake Inhibitors) to help regulate this. Depression tends to run in families and this model holds that some people are more vulnerable to it due to their unique biological factors, such as the presence of depression-triggering genes.

The second school of thought is based on the view that psychosocial factors contribute significantly to depression. These might include prolonged exposure to stressful circumstances, such as failing relationships or excessively demanding work environments. Negative life events, such as losing a job, or traumatic adversities such as sexual, physical and emotional abuse are also common triggers for depression. Treatment here is often based mainly on the talking therapies such as CBT (Cognitive-Behavioural Therapy).

The risk factors for depression are generally grouped into three categories – predisposing, precipitating and perpetuating factors.

Predisposing factors are the pre-existing aspects of your life that increase your risk of developing depression and include your personal history, family background, genetic heritage, upbringing, culture, health, diet and other factors.

Precipitating factors are the psychological and physical triggers that can tip you over into depression, such as stress, illness or a traumatic life event.

Perpetuating factors are the aspects that can maintain the depression such as insomnia or heavy drinking.

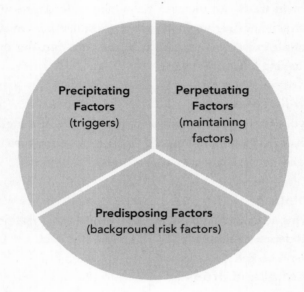

Some of the more common factors that make us vulnerable to depression include:

Stressful life events
It takes time to adjust to traumatic experiences like a death or the breakdown of a significant relationship. Your risk of depression increases if you don't reach out for support.

Physical Illness

You are at higher risk of depression if you suffer from a chronic health condition or have been diagnosed with a serious illness.

Personality

Certain traits can increase vulnerability to depression, such as being overly self-critical, perfectionist, pessimistic, prone to excessive worrying, having a rigid thinking style or having low self-esteem.

Family History

If your parents had depression, then you're at a higher risk of developing it yourself. Certain genes increase the likelihood of depression after a stressful life event.

Isolation

Living an isolated life can increase your risk of loneliness and depression, especially in later life.

Alcohol and drugs

People often use alcohol and drugs to cope when they're down but the sad fact is that alcohol abuse and substance misuse can also be triggers of depression.

Gender

Women are typically diagnosed with depression twice as often as men. Hormonal fluctuations in the menstrual cycle, in pregnancy, around the time of perimenopause (mid-30s to late 40s) and menopause (early 50s) can make women more vulnerable. Other triggers include infertility and childlessness in women who wanted children. Men with depression, on the other hand, are at greater risk of suicide as they often find it harder to acknowledge their vulnerability and reach out for support.

Types of depression

Depression can be chronic or episodic and comes in various degrees of severity. All of the following types of depression can be helped by using positive psychology techniques, but please seek medical guidance if you think you are suffering from any form of depression.

✦ **Subclinical depression** A small number of symptoms are present but not enough for a diagnosis. At this stage treatment is about prevention rather than cure. Using positive psychology tools, such as the ones in this book, will build your resilience and help prevent symptoms from developing further.

✦ **Mild depression** There are enough symptoms for a diagnosis but only minor functional impairment. Recommended treatment is geared toward self-help and might include making lifestyle changes, such as increasing physical activities, or using techniques such as the examples in this book.

✦ **Moderate depression** More symptoms are present and they have a significant impact on daily life. Treatment options are usually focused on psychological therapies, such as counselling, CBT (Cognitive-Behavioural Therapy) and group therapy, as well as self-help practices like the ones in this book.

✦ **Major depression** This is also known as clinical depression or major depressive disorder and has a pronounced effect on functioning, making the activities of daily life near impossible. Anti-depressant drugs are likely to be prescribed which might be complemented with other methods such as those listed above. Please consult your doctor straightaway if you think you fall into this category.

✦ **Bipolar disorder** Formerly known as manic depression, this is characterized by a cycle of highs (hypomania) alternating with the more frequent devastating lows. Cyclothymia is a milder version of bipolar disorder.

✦ **Persistent depressive disorder** This is also known as dysthymia or chronic depression and is a long-lasting, low-grade form of the illness that can persist for years.

✦ **Postnatal depression** This sometimes happens after giving birth as a result of the hormonal and physical changes and the sense of responsibility for a new life.

✦ **Seasonal Affective Disorder (SAD)** Sometimes known as 'winter depression', this is a seasonal form of depression that can set in with the dwindling daylight causing the mood to plummet.

The downward spiral

Depression is often described as a downward spiral, with thoughts, emotions and behaviours spreading and reinforcing each other. Maybe some of the downward spiral patterns detailed in the list below will seem familiar to you.

✦ **The thought/emotion spiral** You're in the grip of negative thoughts, which sends your emotions plummeting. This has the effect of making your thinking even bleaker and your mood sinks lower as a result.

✦ **The social spiral** You feel down so you don't go out much, so there's no distraction from your low mood and you're less likely to reach out for support, so you feel even more down.

✦ **The physical spiral** You're exhausted, your body hurts and this makes you feel low. You can't summon up the energy to do anything physical to give yourself an endorphin lift so your mood spirals further down.

✦ **The pessimistic spiral** You're expecting the worst to happen. As a result you believe that whatever you do won't make much difference to the situation, so you give up. You feel helpless and sink into despair. This is the cycle of 'learned helplessness' that can feed depression (read more about this in Chapter 7, Learning Optimism).

Introducing positive psychology: what is it and how can it help depression?

Positive psychology is a branch of science that appeared at the end of the 20th century to study the positive aspects of human existence. According to Prof Martin Seligman, co-founder of the field, it is the 'scientific study of optimal human functioning', but it is also widely known as the science of happiness, well-being, resilience, strengths, flourishing, positive emotions and optimism, and these descriptions give you an idea of some of its core parts. Positive psychology has evolved into an applied science with the aim of increasing well-being in individuals, families, schools, workplaces, communities and nations. The goal is to help people move up what might be termed the mental health spectrum in order to flourish. In this context to flourish means to have high emotional, psychological and social well-being.

THE MENTAL HEALTH SPECTRUM

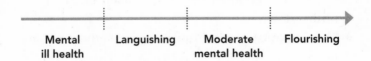

| Mental ill health | Languishing | Moderate mental health | Flourishing |

Every branch of psychology is trying to achieve positive outcomes but the journey to get there is fundamentally different with positive psychology. Mainstream psychology puts the focus on **decreasing mental illness** with the emphasis, for example, on lowering levels of stress and anxiety. Positive psychology, on the other hand, aims directly at **enhancing mental health**, and to *raise* levels of happiness, meaning and satisfaction in life, and this works indirectly to reduce negative functioning.

The Health/Disease Model

Positive psychology operates in the health model (the plus scale) while the mental health profession

DISEASE MODEL	HEALTH MODEL
Depression, Anxiety, Anger, Neurosis	Happiness, Well-being, Satisfaction, Joy
–10 ·········· 0	·········· 10+
Repairing the worst in life	Building the best in life
Focusing on weaknesses	Focusing on strengths
Curing illness	Building well-being
Escaping unhappiness	Increasing happiness
Overcoming deficiencies	Developing competencies
Avoiding pain	Finding enjoyment
Zero as the ceiling	No ceiling

traditionally uses the medical or disease model (the minus scale). The aim in the disease model is to get you from minus (–) to zero (0), that is to say the absence of illness. The *absence* of mental health issues does not, however, equate to the *presence* of well-being and the goal of positive psychology is to go *beyond* zero or neutral into the plus (+) scale and the presence of positive emotions, meaning and other forms of well-being.

Positive psychology interventions are aimed at increasing positive feelings, positive cognitions or positive behaviours. Many of these techniques are common sense. Gratitude, for example, comes from the age-old wisdom of counting your blessings. The difference is that these tools have now been scientifically validated, so we know that they are effective. As such, we call them evidence-based. A major advantage of using these tools is that studies have shown that they not only sustain happiness but, crucially, can also reduce the specific symptoms of depression. They work in both directions to raise and recover well-being. This positive approach heralds a paradigm shift in the way we deal with depression.

The main process used in positive psychology is coaching, which is an action-oriented form of behavioural mentoring. Positive psychology coaching is defined as a scientifically-rooted approach to helping clients increase their well-being, enhance and apply strengths, improve performance and achieve valued goals.[1] It has some clear and specific differences to counselling, which is a form of psychotherapy.

Counselling	Coaching
• Focuses on the past	• Focuses on the future
• 'What is wrong?'	• 'What do you want?'
• Emotional understanding	• Behavioural mentoring
• Looks at pain and difficulty	• Sets goals
• Releases from the past	• Moves forward

Counselling is one of the talking therapies that aims to facilitate an emotional understanding of the source of distress and a cathartic release from the pain. In the 20th century, psychotherapy became widely accepted as the therapy of choice for depression, based on a bold (but largely untested) truism that talking about your troubles is the cure.[2] There's no doubt that for lots of people having a therapist to talk to can be very helpful to gain insight, but for others, including myself, it can actually lead to a worsening of symptoms.[3] My own experience of being in therapy was that going through my traumas over and over again with the therapist kept me trapped in pain rather than getting past it. Research also suggests that the positive changes that occur in some therapy are more likely to be the result of the relationship with the therapist than the therapy itself.[4]

What the therapeutic process lacked was a focus on overall holistic well-being but I'm pleased to say that this is changing. One positive approach to therapy is 'positive psychotherapy' (PPT), developed by some of the leading researchers in the field, which combines the practice of psychotherapy with positive psychology interventions. According to Dr Tayyab Rashid who, with Prof Martin Seligman, pioneered the field of positive psychology, accentuating positive resources may serve clients best not when life is easy but when life gets difficult. Rather than concentrating on your weaknesses, positive psychology sessions focus on harnessing your strengths, so you can use them as a toolkit to work toward improving what is good in your life. Session themes include positive emotions, gratitude, savouring, strengths, meaning and relationships, which are all also chapters in this book. The idea behind this and other forms of positive therapy is that enhancing well-being and building up a client's positive resources will often automatically weaken or eliminate many of the factors that can maintain depression, such as pessimism or low self-confidence.

In my practice as a positive psychologist over the years I've seen these tools working well both in coaching and groupwork. One of the most memorable occasions was when I designed a pilot intervention called The Happiness Zones, for alcohol-misusing adolescents.[5] The teens were in the habit of using drinking as a quick release from the stress they were under, to escape from their many problems and as a shortcut to get happy. They lacked stability – most were in temporary accommodation, estranged from their families, living in hostels or 'sofa-surfing' with friends. Their problems were wide-ranging – finances, literacy, violence, drugs, abuse, crime, health and family breakdown. Most had dropped out of education and one teenager was pregnant. All of them were deep into the minus scale (*see* p13). None of them felt they had any hope for the future.

Instead of taking the conventional 'disease model' approach of focusing on their problem drinking, those issues were put to one side, with only one of the eight sessions directly addressing alcohol misuse. Instead, the course concentrated on well-being, with sessions on happiness, positive emotions, optimism, resilience, meditation, strengths, positive relationships, goal-setting and the body–mind connection.

This turned out to be a surprisingly successful approach. As the weeks went by the young people started feeling better. And the positive changes that were happening on the inside were mirrored on the outside. Most of the group went back into education, there were new jobs and homes, relationships were repaired, there was calm in place of the usual chaos and a noticeably improved vitality. It all amounted to a transformation. One of the most promising outcomes of this focus on well-being was that the drinking dropped dramatically, with some of the group giving up alcohol altogether. And all this was achieved simply by parking those very problems!

The Happiness Zones went on to be named as an example of best practice in mental well-being by the Academy of Social Sciences in the UK.[6] I have since used the Zones as the basis for other positive psychology programmes that I've developed for a variety of groups.

Incidentally, the pregnant teenager, whose pessimism was such that her key worker described her as 'almost afraid to think of what good can happen for fear of what bad might happen', went on to give birth to a beautiful daughter and named her… Faith.

Turning to you

Whether you're at risk of depression or already experiencing the reality of it, positive psychology offers tried and tested practices that can both prevent depression and help to cure it. These are tools that you can draw on to build your own resilience to depression – a bit like pulling on a warm sweater to protect you from the cold. Although they may be easier to engage with at the mild-to-moderate end of the depression spectrum, they are useful at every stage of recovery. Positive psychotherapy (PPT), for example, has been used with severely-depressed individuals as a supplement to traditional methods of treatment, and was found to relieve symptoms of depression and lead to more remission than either drug treatment or their usual treatment alone.[7]

The key thing to remember is the importance of practice. Neuroscience has shown us that the brain has a high degree of neuroplasticity – that is to say it is quite malleable and can be rewired over time. Your brain is shaped by life events but can also be reshaped by training it. The more a technique is practised the more connections are made and strengthened in the brain.

Taking small steps leads to positive neural changes and has a cumulative effect. The practice of gratitude (*see* Chapter 4), for example, produces serotonin, which leads to an improved mood, which might then motivate you to further positive action. This can trigger an upward spiral out of depression.

A metaphor that many of my clients have found helpful is to think of your well-being as a lake or reservoir on which you are sailing. There are huge boulders in the water signifying the rocky times in life. If the water level of your resilience is low, you are more likely to wreck your boat on these rocks. But if you feed your reservoir with positive actions, positive emotions and optimistic thinking, the level of your resilience will rise and you'll be better able to sail right over those rocks. You are cushioned against adversity. One of the founders of positive psychology, Prof Chris Peterson, once said memorably that 'Happiness is not a spectator sport'. If you want to grow your happiness you have to go beyond intellectual curiosity and put your knowledge into action. That's why reading this book is only part of the journey. What will really make the difference is applying the practices.

How to use this book

This book offers you a positive approach to overcome depression using scientifically-grounded practices that work as natural anti-depressants. The text is supplemented by comprehensive chapter notes that can be found at the back of the book. Specifically the practices presented can:

+ Improve your mood
+ Prevent depression
+ Reduce depression symptoms
+ Relieve residual symptoms of major depression
+ Prevent relapse into depression
+ Build resilience
+ Increase happiness and well-being
+ Complement other forms of depression treatment

You can practise these techniques as self-help or alongside other treatment methods, and I recommend that you check in with your doctor or mental health practitioner for guidance. This is especially vital if you have been experiencing suicidal thoughts.

Depression is a mental disorder that affects emotions, thinking, the body and how we interact with others, and this is reflected in the range of chapters in this book which address these aspects of well-being. Approach your self-management of depression by trying a variety of the strategies suggested to see which work best for you. Most of them are based on building positives. For some people this will seem counter-intuitive and too indirect – why mess around with happiness tools when the problem is depression? But if you focus on activities that grow well-being, the research suggests your well-being will grow.

Remember that depression shrinks what you think you're capable of and keeps you trapped in lowness. This is about trying something different. You are the best guide as to what will work well for you, so trust your instincts on this. You are more likely to persist with a technique if you are instinctively drawn to using it.

Here are some other tips on using the positive psychology techniques in this book for success.

Adopt a 'growth mindset'

Do you believe that your abilities are set in stone (a fixed mindset) or that you can become better at most things if you put in the effort (a growth mindset)? These two mindsets influence our potential to develop, according to leading Stanford researcher Prof Carol Dweck, author of *Mindset*.[8]

Someone with a **fixed mindset** believes that we are born with a certain amount of abilities that are more or less fixed at birth. So, if something goes wrong, say a relationship fails, we can end up labelling ourselves as no good at relationships and lose self-esteem. A fixed mindset makes it more likely that we will feel depressed when a setback occurs, respond in a helpless way and give up.

Someone in a **growth mindset**, on the other hand, believes that with enough motivation, concentration and application we can become better at most things we put our minds to. This mindset views failure as feedback and a lesson to take forward for the next time around.

The growth mindset is one of the foundations in positive psychology – a belief that we can learn optimism, grow our happiness and develop our strengths. It is a compassionate mindset to have when working at making a change. Try something and if it doesn't work out, remember that this is your feedback to be flexible – have another go later or try something new. Adopting a growth mindset makes it easier to venture out of your comfort zone and experiment without beating yourself up if it's not perfect first time.

One thing a day

Depression is a profoundly draining experience and when it strikes it can be very hard to summon up the energy to do anything at all. That's why it's a good idea to be realistic about your expectations and aim to do one small thing a day, even if this is just walking to the shops. It's still a nudge in the right direction. Remember to be kind to yourself. You can always try to do more but don't beat yourself up if this turns out to be unsustainable. Think small steps.

Know your preferences

If you're normally quite a sociable person, then make a plan to do something you know you've enjoyed doing before, such as arranging to meet up with an old friend.

Also, if you want to vary how you work with a particular practice – go ahead. Variety is the spice of life so, if you get bored see if you can invent your own twist on a technique to keep it fresh or make it a better fit for you.

Stretch yourself

Try something new. You may be pleasantly surprised when you venture out of your comfort zone.

+ If you're the kind of person who spends a lot of time 'in your head' you might try one of the positive emotions' techniques (*see* Chapter 3) or the physical activities in the chapter on Vitality (*see* Chapter 10).

+ If you're overwhelmed by emotions, why not try addressing your thinking habits with the tools in the Learning Optimism chapter (*see* p107) or distracting yourself by doing something practical from the chapter on Positive Directions (*see* p209).

It's all about the reps

Finally, like any form of training, mind training requires regular repetition to make a habit out of the practice. So, the more you train your brain to tune into the positive things in life, the easier and more automatic this becomes.

It would be unrealistic to imagine that you can make the transition from depression to happiness in one big leap. Rather look on it as taking incremental steps. Also remember that the nature of happiness is not a permanent state. Those top-of-the-range emotions like bliss, elation and ecstasy are only ever transitory experiences even when *not* suffering from depression. The aim is not so much to chase those momentary highs but to invest in raising your underlying level of well-being, which is a more realistic prospect. Try to do more of the things that leave you feeling a little bit better. It is the multiplicity of small positive actions that will help you on the road to recovery.

The ones to read

Second Wave Positive Psychology by Itai Ivtzan, Tim Lomas, Kate Hefferon and Piers Worth

The Upward Spiral by Alex Korb

CHAPTER 2

The Science of Happiness

I'D LIKE TO SHARE WITH YOU some of the story of positive psychology as the scientific study of happiness and a few of the models it has generated. This will give you some clues as to what might be missing from your own well-being. Psychology had three broad aims in the first half of the 20th century – to cure mental illness, to nurture high talent and to improve people's lives. But after the trauma of the Second World War, the science narrowed its scope to the first of these. This led to great progress being made in alleviating the suffering caused by mental illness, but what it meant was that the positive aspects of life – such as what gives life meaning and what it takes to flourish – became neglected areas of research. Instead, psychology began to view people more as passive victims of their internal pathological drives, damaged brains or external stressors. We were left with an unbalanced science which had become a psychology of the negative, focusing most of its research into people's deficits, highlighting shortcomings over strengths.

Positive psychology emerged as a new branch of science in the late 1990s as an attempt to rebalance the field and apply the scientific method to questions such as what it takes for us to feel good and function well. This has led to an abundance of research in areas of well-being, such as happiness, positive emotions, strengths, optimism, hope, flow, mindfulness, love, wisdom, meaning, courage, creativity, authenticity, motivation and goals. The science has built on the foundations of its direct ancestor, humanistic psychology, which similarly eschewed the what-is-wrong-with-people approach to focus instead on human potential, growth, fulfilment and self-actualization. Although it has the positive tag, this doesn't mean that the science of well-being doesn't 'do' negative or that it ignores or denies the difficult aspects of life. In fact there is one area of the science – post-traumatic growth – that is about the unexpected positives that can emerge from life's most negative events. Positive psychology deals with the negatives in life by looking at positive ways of coping and through exploring areas such as resilience – how to bounce back from tough times and thrive in periods of adversity.

This branch of psychology was co-founded by Professor Martin Seligman, author of *Learned Optimism*, *Authentic Happiness* and *Flourish*, alongside Prof Mihaly Csikszentmihalyi, who put the study of 'flow' on the map. Seligman's own career has paralleled the transition in psychology from studying the negative to the positive, from 'learned helplessness' to 'learned optimism'. At the heart of the field has been the study of 'subjective well-being', the scientific term for happiness that reflects the personal way in which we rate our well-being. We now know a lot more about the anatomy of happiness, what it is and how to achieve it. Researchers have come up with a number of formulae, some of which are discussed below. These models will give you clues as to what it will take to restore your well-being.

The Happiness Formula

Around 40 percent of your happiness is under your direct voluntary control and can be increased by the activities you engage in and your outlook on life.[1] So, regardless of the hand you've been dealt in life, there is a lot you can do to influence your level of happiness.

$$H = S + C + V^2$$

H is your enduring level of happiness. Think of it as your baseline level of contentment rather than being about transient positive emotions such as joy.

S is your biological set point. This is determined by genes and accounts for around 50 percent of your happiness.

Whether you have a significant positive or negative life event, you will gradually revert to your set range.

C is for your circumstances or conditions in life. This accounts for only 10 percent of your happiness, which is probably less than you might imagine. So, changing your circumstances, such as going for a better job or moving to a new house, will only have a marginal effect on your happiness, although this tends to be where we focus our efforts.

V is the part that's under voluntary control and it accounts for around 40 percent of your happiness. So nearly half of our happiness can be influenced by the activities we engage in, such as the positive psychology practices described in this book.

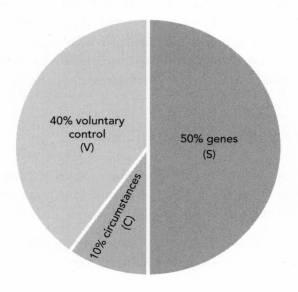

Happiness is ...

Martin Seligman identified three main pathways to authentic happiness,[3] which will help you work out where you seek yours and what, if anything, might be out of balance.

Pleasure is about the feel-good factor, enjoyment, positive emotions and energy.

Engagement is about how engaged you are with life – with work, people, activities. It also refers to flow – being 'in the zone'.

Meaning is about the things you value that give your life meaning and purpose.

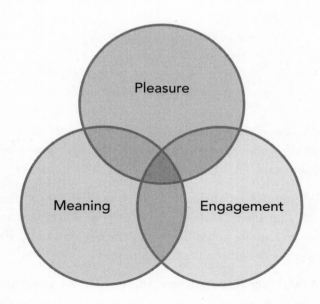

PERMA[4]

The pleasure–engagement–meaning model of authentic happiness was broadened in 2011 into the PERMA model to incorporate some of the other ingredients of flourishing. Each of these pathways to well-being is featured in this book.

✦ Positive emotion
✦ Engagement
✦ Relationships
✦ Meaning
✦ Accomplishment

$$SWB \text{ (Subjective Well-Being)} = SWL + \text{high PA} + \text{low NA}^{5}$$

This formula for Subjective Well-Being combines how you think about happiness (cognitive) with how you feel (emotional).

SWL stands for Satisfaction With Life. Are you satisfied with your life or is there a gap between where you are now and where you'd like to be. The bigger the gap the lower you will be on life satisfaction.

PA (high) stands for Positive Affect and refers to the sum of your experience of positive emotions. This is about the frequency with which you experience positive emotions rather than the intensity.

NA (low) is Negative Affect, the sum of your experience of negative emotions. Subjective Well-Being requires the quantity of positive affect to be higher than negative affect.

Psychological well-being[6]

There are six elements in this model of well-being. If you can put a tick in each of these domains, then you are experiencing psychological well-being. If you are low in any of these areas, then that is a clue as to where to apply your focus.

✦ Self-acceptance – accepting yourself for who you are
✦ Positive relationships – having quality connections to others
✦ Life purpose – having meaningful goals and direction in life
✦ Personal growth – fostering ongoing growth and personal development
✦ Autonomy – having a sense of personal control in thought and action
✦ Environmental mastery – managing your life and surroundings effectively

Flow[7]

Flow is a form of engagement, a state of absorption where you're so immersed in an enjoyable activity that you may lose track of time. You feel completely at one with what you're doing – in the moment – and it's generally after the experience that you appreciate the pleasure it brings. Flow in itself is a neutral state. What puts you into flow is often related to your interests, whether creative, sporty, educational, vocational or spiritual. Reading, dancing, gardening, making music, jogging and cookery are frequently mentioned as flow-inducers. When coaching clients say that positive emotions feel out of reach, I often suggest that they try a flow activity instead.

Self-determination theory[8]

This model suggests that we have three fundamental needs for well-being.

✦ **Autonomy** – a sense of control over what you do
✦ **Competence** – feeling confident in what you do
✦ **Relatedness** – having close, secure connections

Short-term or sustainable happiness?

By now you'll have realized that there is more than one form of well-being and an abundance of routes to it, thankfully! Essentially, well-being can be divided into one of two types:

✦ **Hedonic well-being** is the better-known form of happiness. It is the feel-good factor of pleasure, a cheerful mood and positive emotions such as joy. You'll recognize this as peak happiness.

✦ **Eudaimonic well-being** (*see* p211) is an umbrella term that refers to a deeper happiness of meaning and purpose and how you are at your best, playing to your strengths and realizing your potential. Think of it as your baseline of contentment.

A happy balance

Happiness is about finding the balance of pleasure (hedonic well-being) and purpose (eudaimonic well-being) that is right for you and will give you the most fulfilled life. The trouble with pleasure is that it leads to a short-term high that is concentrated but fades fast. That's because we have a 'hedonic treadmill'; we adapt to the things that give us pleasure and begin to take them for granted, so they stop working as well. The second time you eat at that fantastic restaurant is never as good as the first time. After a while your new car fails to give you the thrill it once did. Engagement and meaning are pathways to eudaimonic well-being, which is a longer-lasting and therefore more sustainable happiness than the peaks and troughs of hedonic well-being.

Your life map

Take a look at your own life now and note your balance between Pleasure, Engagement (Flow) and Meaning. Choose a time span, maybe the last 24 hours or the last week. How did you spend your time? Think back over your activities and list them in the left-hand column of the chart opposite. Then decide which category, if any, they fall into Pleasure, Engagement or Meaning. Ask yourself these questions:

✦ What is the balance like between the three categories?
✦ Is the balance how you would like it to be?
✦ Do you need more, less or the same amount of time for pleasure, engagement or meaning?
✦ What actions could you take to achieve a better balance?

By doing this you'll begin to get a sense of whether the balance in your life is toward the short high of hedonic well-being (pleasure) or the deeper fulfilment of eudaimonic well-being (engagement and meaning), and whether this is right for you or not.

ACTIVITY	TYPE OF HAPPINESS			
	Pleasure	Engagement (Flow)	Meaning	None of these

The facts and fiction of happiness

New research is emerging all the time from the science of happiness. Let's bust some of the common myths that can hold us back in our quest for personal contentment. Here's the lowdown on what does and doesn't make us happy.

Makes us happy?	Fact	Fiction
Wealth		✘ Once there's enough money to cover the necessities of life, money ceases to have much impact on our well-being.
Love and connections	✔ Relationships and being actively social are major sources of happiness.	
Education		✘ Your level of education has little impact although it leads to opportunities.
Work	✔ Engaging work and job satisfaction count.	
Youth		✘ Happiness does not lessen with age. There's a low point around the 40s–early 50s but then it rises again.

Makes us happy?	Fact	Fiction
Physical well-being	✔ Sleep, exercise and diet affect your mood.	
Beauty		✘ Being attractive does not lead to greater happiness.
Spirituality	✔ Engaging in some form of spiritual practice has benefits.	
Living in a sunny climate		✘ Sunshine and warmth only have a marginal impact on your level of happiness.
Health	✔ What you think about your state of health has an effect (subjective) …	✘ … but your *actual* health (objective) has little connection to your happiness, except in the case of serious illness.
Children	✔ Having children gives your life meaning (eudaimonic well-being) …	✘ … but lowers hedonic well-being, especially where the toddler and teen years are concerned.

The paradox of happiness

For such a desirable goal (happiness is enshrined in the American Constitution as an inalienable right), pursuing it is a haphazard affair. In my own experience I've found that making happiness the goal is more likely to backfire, as it slips in and out of your hands. To paraphrase John Lennon, happiness seems to happen while you're busy making other plans. Happiness is best regarded as a by-product of attempts to raise your well-being. The pressure to be happy can backfire and create an extra burden for people who are already suffering. There is some evidence to suggest that when you set happiness itself as the goal, you're likely to have unrealistically high standards and to be disappointed when you fail to reach those heights or stay up there.[9] It is far better to set a low goal – aim for a feeling of satisfaction rather than the peak of happiness. As many of the positive psychology models show, there is a lot more to happiness than feeling good. Savour the positive moments as and when they occur – but suspend any judgment over whether you're feeling happier or not. Keep a light touch about raising your level of happiness and remember that those highs are transient. Enjoy them in the moment, but don't cling onto them. And remember that the pursuit of happiness is much broader than the pursuit of pleasure. There are all those activities that bring meaning, purpose and engagement into life.

In the next chapter we look at one of the major players in the recovery from depression – positive emotions –

with the chapters that follow detailing the techniques that will raise your experience of positivity.

The ones to read

Authentic Happiness and *Flourish*, both by Martin Seligman

Flow by Mihaly Csikszentmihalyi

The How of Happiness by Sonja Lyubomirsky

Positive Psychology in a Nutshell by Ilona Boniwell

The Happiness Training Plan by Miriam Akhtar and Dr Chris Johnstone (www.happinesstrainingplan.com)

Positive Psychology News Daily (www.positivepsychologynews.com)

CHAPTER 3

Positive Emotions: The Upward Spiral to Well-being

+ **What is it about?** Positive emotions play a key role in the positive approach to depression.
+ **In other words:** They not only feel good, they do us good, too.
+ **Try this for:** Boosting mood naturally, happiness, resilience and well-being.

> *A joyful heart is good medicine*
> Book of Proverbs

Ah, the joy of positive emotions … so elevating and yet so elusive in depression! They might bubble up through that loving connection you have with someone or in that quiet space of peace and contemplation; when you are inspired by a new idea or awestruck by the beauty of nature. Positive emotions may be fleeting, but these good feelings play a vital role in well-being and the recovery from depression. There is a power in positive emotions that goes beyond the pleasure in the moment. One of the major discoveries in positive psychology is that positive emotions not only feel good, they do us good, too. They help us to feel better, bolster us against life's stresses and stimulate us to recover from adversity and access an upward spiral of emotional well-being, which counteracts the downward spiral into depression.

Positive emotions hold the key to the positive psychology approach to depression. I experienced how well this works in my own journey out of depression. I spent years exploring my negative emotions in therapy, digging deep into my unhappiness, re-opening wounds and bringing past hurt to the front of my mind. But it wasn't until I went down the opposite route, building my experience of positive emotions that I finally began to recover and move out of depression. In the following chapters you'll find many practices that increase positivity.

The role of emotions

Emotions reflect the complex nature of being human. You can experience both positive and negative emotions at the same time – joy tinged with sadness, for example. Emotions tend to be short-lived and triggered by something specific whereas moods are longer-lasting and are more free-floating rather than being the direct consequence of something.

Our emotions act as signals, our internal guidance system. A negative emotion, such as fear or anger, tells us something is wrong and needs fixing, whereas a positive emotion lets us know that something good is happening and we're on track toward our hopes and goals.

Negative emotions alert us to danger, sending out a warning that something needs to be fixed. These emotions prompt us into specific actions. They activate the 'fight or flight' response of the body's survival instinct. Anger leads to attack, fear to escape. The prehistoric family, faced with a large mammal charging toward them, would experience fear, prompting them to flee. The same still holds true today. Faced with a runaway car hurtling toward you, fear will propel you to get out of the way. Negative emotions narrow our thinking, so that we can tackle the immediate threat to our well-being. They are powerful experiences.

I remember the day I moved into a room above a café, when I was a student living in France. My neighbour seemed friendly and showed me around the place. Late that night there was a knock at the door. I opened it and to my horror the neighbour was standing there wearing nothing but his birthday suit...! In that moment of sheer terror, I managed to shove a heavy wardrobe across the door. I trembled all night until I heard the café owner arrive in the morning to open up downstairs. It was then that I went to move the wardrobe. Only I found it really hard to shift, whereas during the night the emotion of fear had given me the presence of mind and strength to spot the wardrobe's potential to shield me and move it in a flash. This illustrates how negative emotions can work for us. They narrow our thought–action repertoires to those that best suit our survival in threatening situations.

Negative emotions are naturally in abundance when suffering from depression and can be overwhelming. It may be some consolation to know that there is also a positive purpose to these painful feelings.

Sadness can act as a form of self-preservation, helping us to disengage from harmful situations and hibernate to recover our strength.

Anxiety is an early warning system that sweeps the environment for threats and initiates defence strategies to avert a crisis or lessen the effects of a negative event.

Loneliness is the shadow side of solitude. It can reveal aspects of our wants and needs that get overlooked when we're in company.

Anger is a moral emotion that can motivate us to put right a wrong.

Guilt is also a form of condemnation, but of ourselves rather than something external. This can help us become better people by accepting responsibility for a misdeed and be a motivating force to live a better life.

Negative emotions are bigger experiences than positive emotions, even when there is no immediate threat involved. They also last longer – they hang around and weigh you down, whereas positive emotions are much lighter, more fleeting experiences. In the past, psychology research was largely focused on studying negative emotions and not much was known about the purpose of these short-lived good feelings. That was until Prof Barbara Fredrickson, principal investigator of the PEPLab (Positive Emotions and Psychophysiology Lab) at the University of North Carolina, emerged as the world's leading researcher on positive emotions.

What positive emotions can do for you

Barbara Fredrickson has discovered that there are benefits to experiencing positive emotions that go far beyond feeling good. Positive emotions open up our hearts and minds to new ideas and experiences. Whereas negative emotions narrow and focus our thinking, positive emotions broaden our thinking and over time they accumulate to build multiple resources that support our well-being. Fredrickson named this the broaden-and-build theory of positive emotions.[1]

POSITIVE EMOTIONS

Past	Present	Future
Contentment	Love	Hope
Satisfaction	Awe	Optimism
Fulfilment	Joy	Faith
Pride	Bliss	Trust
Serenity	Ecstasy	Excitement
Gratitude	Inspiration	
	Calm	
	Peace	
	Pleasure	
	Curiosity	
	Interest	
	Amusement	
	Creativity	

Broaden the mind

Positive emotions broaden our thinking and the scope of our attention, and prompt us into a wide range of action. They make us more open-minded, creative and flexible thinkers, capable of big-picture thinking. If you want to generate new ideas or find a creative solution, you might be better off doing something that makes you feel good rather than stressing your way to the answer. Positive emotions broaden our thought–action repertoires.

+ **Joy** leads to an urge to play, to push the limits and be creative.
+ **Interest** causes a desire to seek out new information, to explore the world and expand the self.
+ **Contentment** is a prompt to savour and integrate new perspectives into your world.
+ **Pride** makes you think big.
+ **Elevation** inspires you to become better.
+ **Love** makes you want to share and explore with others, plus all of the above.

Build up resources

Although short-lived in themselves, positive emotions accumulate to produce long-lasting personal resources that we can draw on at other times.

+ **Psychological resources** Positive emotions help develop optimism and resilience. They also shape your sense of identity and create the motivation to pursue goals.
+ **Intellectual resources** Positive emotions develop problem-solving skills and assist with learning new information.
+ **Social resources** Positive emotions help you form new relationships and deepen the bonds of existing ones.
+ **Physical resources** Positive emotions help you develop co-ordination, strength and cardiovascular health.

Some of these benefits, such as positive emotions building physical resources, may surprise you. However, if you're feeling curious, for example, you're more likely to explore the world around you and this leads to greater physical activity, which builds fitness, muscle, etc.

Speed recovery from negative emotions

If you're suffering from stress positive emotions are particularly relevant. Experiments have shown how positive emotions can undo the ill-effects that negatives have on the body – such as increasing blood pressure and raising heart rate – and help it return to homeostasis, a state of equilibrium. A feeling of contentment or amusement, for example, speeds the physical recovery from stress. Barbara Fredrickson calls this your hidden 'reset' button. When you're faced with a stressful situation, you can't stop your heart from beating harder, but positivity will help to rein in those cardiovascular reactions and regain a calm heart.[2] In her experiments Fredrickson showed people film clips that evoked positive emotions such as serenity and amusement, which led to a faster recovery from the after-effects of stress than when they were shown negative or neutral clips. This is something you can easily do for yourself when you experience stress – watch a comedy, for instance, or listen to some calming or uplifting music.

Positive emotions protect you from depression and can stop you relapsing. The more positivity you experience, the greater your ability to cope with adversity. To return to the metaphor introduced in Chapter 1, it's like filling a reservoir so that your level of well-being is higher and consequently your resilience is strengthened, so that you're in a better position to survive the crisis. (*See* Chapter 8, Resilience.)

The upward spiral

So far we've discussed some of the roles that positive emotions play in broadening the mind, building up personal resources and dissolving the effects of negativity. All of these are beneficial in depression – to help you think flexibly when you might be in a fixed mindset, to give you resources to draw on when you're at your most vulnerable and to up your resilience so you're better able to keep going. The next step out of depression is to increase the ratio of positive emotions you experience in order to trigger the upward spiral and get onto the path to flourishing. I've witnessed many times in my coaching practice, and from my own experience, how when you feel better, life seems to go better too. In fact, there is a virtuous circle between happiness and success. You feel happy when something goes right but the opposite is also true too. When you feel good things are more likely to go well. Success leads to happiness AND happiness leads to success. This is the upward spiral in action creating a new cycle of growth, which can culminate in a personal transformation. I saw it happen in the work I did with teenagers in the Happiness Zones (*see* p16). As they began to feel better, changes occurred and life took a definite turn for the better with problems resolved and improved circumstances. The transformation was visible even in the way they looked – they had more vitality, clearer skin and were better dressed! You may recognize this from your own life – special times when everything you touched seemed to be working well.

Growing your positivity

So how do you increase your experience of positive emotions? It helps to know something more about the way these feelings operate. Positive emotions generally arise as a result of the things we do, the way we see the world and how we interpret the events in our lives. When you notice the good stuff, what's right in your life rather than what's wrong, or do something that's meaningful for you, you'll be cultivating a positive emotion. You will really need to tune in against the competition of 'louder' negative emotions, however. Approach this with a lightness of touch, be open to the experience and remain relaxed about the outcome. Do the practice but let go of the result – accept that positive emotions are transient and somewhat unpredictable. Sometimes it will work, sometimes it won't. Here are a few tips to get you started on the upward spiral.

✦ Ask yourself: 'What's going right in my life right now?' What is there to be pleased with? To be grateful for?'

✦ Identify what you love doing and do more of it. What puts sunshine into your soul? A spring into your step? What makes your heart sing rather than sink? Who do you love to be around?

✦ Engage wholeheartedly with a positive experience in the moment – without analyzing it. (This is the surest way of deflating your experience.)

✦ Focus on quantity rather than the quality of positive emotions. It is frequency rather than intensity of emotion that counts. Experiencing lots of mildly positive emotions like curiosity and calm will enhance your well-being more than those rarer experiences like bliss.

✦ Equally, remember that you'll never get rid of negative emotions altogether. They are entirely natural reactions and it would not be desirable to eradicate them. Negative emotions have a function and provide the contrast so that you can truly appreciate the positive when it happens.

Don't try to 'fake it until you make it'. Feigning positive emotions to cover up negativity can lead to a toxic insincerity that puts the body under stress. You're aiming for an authentic, heartfelt positivity, grounded in reality rather than something forced, fake or trivial. On the opposite page is a Positive Emotions kit list showing some of the evidence-based tools that increase positivity. I like to think of them as items in a kitbag. It's useful to carry as many of them around as possible. A variety of these practices are featured in the chapters that follow.

P.E. (Positive Emotions) kit

✦ Gratitude
✦ Savouring
✦ Acts of kindness
✦ Connecting with loved ones
✦ Using your strengths
✦ Mindfulness meditation
✦ Loving-kindness meditation
✦ Physical activity
✦ Visualizing your future positively (a practice known as Best Possible Self)

Barbara Fredrickson recommends finding out what makes you feel truly alive and to give those activities a higher priority. A lot of this is about prioritizing time to play, love and enjoy. In the time-crunched era we live in, where we're expected to be on call 24/7, space to play is increasingly rare as adults. However, given the benefits of tapping into positive emotions, especially knowing that this is also a route to flourishing, isn't it worth dedicating some time to it?

A playlist

In the same way that you might put together a play-list of your favourite tracks on an MP3 player, one idea to increase the frequency of your positive emotional experiences is to put together a list of things you enjoy doing and then commit to doing some of them on a regular basis. Recreational activities are ways to have fun, to explore something new and to put life's trials to one side. Try to do something at least once daily, if only for a quarter of an hour. Make sure it's something you can access easily. Active recreation, such as gardening or taking part in pub quizzes, is more satisfying and rewarding than passive leisure such as watching TV. Remember, it is the quantity of positive emotional experiences that counts. When I first did this, some of the things I had on my list included walks in the park, dancing *le roc* (French jive), meeting up with friends, going to perfume shops to smell all the lovely scents and visiting new cafés. Compile a list of some of your favourite activities and schedule something from your playlist to do every day.

PLAYLIST – THINGS I ENJOY ...

1. ....

....

2. ....

....

3. ....

....

4. ....

....

5. ....

....

6. ....

....

Based on *Quality of Life Therapy*[3]

Here's one final thought to inspire you to give yourself permission to enjoy life.

> By investing in activities that generate positive emotions, you're investing in your future and opening yourself up to the possibility of a transformation.

The ones to read
Positivity by Barbara Fredrickson
The Positive Power of Negative Emotions by Tim Lomas

CHAPTER 4

The Attitude of Gratitude

✦ **What is it?** A feeling of thankfulness, wonder and appreciation for life.
✦ **Try this for:** Positive emotions, happiness, satisfaction with life, relationships, as a cure for envy and disillusionment.
✦ **If you like this, try also:** Savouring the Moment (Chapter 5), Meditation (Chapter 6).

The author Sarah Ban Breathnach brought the 'gratitude journal' to international attention when she appeared on *The Oprah Winfrey Show* in the 1990s and introduced a worldwide television audience to the idea of keeping a diary of the good things in life.[1] I was one of those watching and I have kept a gratitude journal ever since. Many journal keepers describe it as life-changing; it was for me. It was the key to switching from a mindset of scarcity, aware of what was lacking in my life, to one of abundance, appreciative of all the many good things I have.

You may have grown up being told to 'count your blessings'. Well, it turns out that wisdom was spot on. The evidence suggests that gratitude is one of the most powerful practices you can use to raise your well-being, described by Prof Sonja Lyubomirsky of the University of California at Riverside as a kind of meta-strategy for achieving happiness.[2] It all comes from asking simple questions like: 'What is good in my life?' 'What am I grateful for?' and 'What went well?'

Gratitude is much more than saying thank you. It's about tuning in and noticing the positives, training the mind to see how the glass is more full than empty. Our brains have a natural tendency to pay more attention to the negative. We spot what's wrong before we notice what's right. So when a child comes home clutching their school report, the parent's attention is drawn to the D they got in history before registering the As in science and geography. This 'negativity bias' is one of the barriers to happiness and is intensified in depression. When you're down you notice more negatives about yourself and the world around you, pulling your mood further down.

Practising gratitude is an antidote to the negativity bias and has a wide range of benefits for well-being. These range from positive emotions to happiness, satisfaction with life, good self-esteem, optimism, hope, enthusiasm, empathy, vitality, spirituality and forgiveness. In *The How of Happiness* Prof Sonja Lyubomirsky identifies eight ways that gratitude builds happiness.[3]

✦ Encourages the savouring of positive life experiences
✦ Boosts self-esteem
✦ Helps you to cope with stress and adjust to difficult circumstances
✦ Deters negative emotions
✦ Promotes positive behaviour
✦ Nurtures relationships and reduces the likelihood of making unfavourable social comparisons to people you think are better off
✦ Mitigates against hedonic adaptation, where we take the good things in life for granted
✦ Leads to greater engagement with physical activity and fewer bodily ailments

Higher levels of gratitude are, crucially, linked to lower levels of depression, anxiety, loneliness, envy, neuroticism and materialism. Gratitude can act as a remedy for rumination, a feature of depression where the mind obsesses endlessly over negative events and personal failings.[4] It also acts as protection in cases of high levels of hopelessness, a risk factor for suicide.

Gratitude is appreciation of what we have. Prof Robert Emmons of the University of California, Davis, the foremost researcher on gratitude, describes it as a two-stage process: firstly, acknowledging what is good in our life; secondly recognizing that the source of it lies at least partially outside ourselves. In essence, it is an appreciation of something external, an awareness of the benefits that we are not responsible for ourselves but are still fortunate to have, and this makes us grateful. With depression, gratitude helps in three major ways, which Emmons refers to as the ARC model of gratitude.

Gratitude amplifies: Like a loudspeaker, gratitude increases the volume of good in our lives. The good that we see in ourselves, in others and the world is multiplied. It is the counterpart to the negativity bias.

Gratitude rescues: We are exposed to a constant drip of negativity, whether from our own internal thoughts and negative situations or to the daily news headlines of doom and gloom that spread the fear factor. When we are emotionally exhausted and weighed down by this negativity, we need to hear good news. Gratitude is the best weapon to counter these internal and external threats that rob us of sustainable joy.

Gratitude connects: Kindness is what keeps communities functioning well. Without gratitude these relationships would unravel. Gratitude is the all-purpose glue that bonds people, strengthening and solidifying relationships. Without gratitude societies would crumble.

By feeling grateful, we are acknowledging that someone, somewhere, is being kind to us. That we are worthy of receiving kindness and that it does exist in the world and, therefore, that life may be worth living.

Gratitude Tools

With my coaching clients I always make the point that growing your happiness is about putting the knowledge you've gained into practice. Intellectual curiosity will only get you so far, it's the regular use of positive psychology techniques and practices that will make a sustainable difference to your well-being. That isn't easy when you're in the midst of depression but it might help to know that just by doing the practice you are developing new neural connections, which become stronger with repetition like a forest path becomes more evident each time someone walks along it. Gratitude also stimulates production of two feel-good neurotransmitters – dopamine and serotonin. The practice that started me on the upward spiral out of depression was:

'Three Good Things'

This is about counting blessings rather than burdens. It doesn't require material wealth but more an attitude of thankfulness regardless of current circumstances. Think of three specific things that are good in your life, that you are grateful for or that have gone well for you. It could be a big thing such as a place to call your own or something small like finding a parking space next to the entrance. It could be a special friend or something as simple as eating a delicious apple. It can be hard to think of anything that's gone well in depression so stick to noticing the small achievements, such as managing to make a phone call or send an email. Celebrate the progress too. If you are able to do a complete circuit of the park whereas before you only walked half the distance, then this is something to include on your list. This exercise can be done at any time – on your commute to work, while walking the dog or anchored to a routine like brushing your teeth. People often do it at bedtime to reflect on the day that's been, which results in improved sleep and feeling more refreshed on waking up.

Of course when you're down it is a struggle to see any positives but if you look hard enough you will find something to be thankful for, whether it is living in a safe area or having two legs that can get you from A to B. I tend to fall back on expressing gratitude for my home as the system that looks after my needs. I appreciate the pipes that bring in gas and water, the roof that keeps me dry, the walls that keep me warm, the electricity that powers the house, the broadband that keeps me connected, the computer that enables me to work from home, the view that inspires me and the neighbours who look out for me.

This technique works by stimulating positive emotions, so that we *feel* grateful rather than just thinking gratitude. It can feel like a dry little exercise at first and it certainly took me a while before doing gratitude in my head translated into a heart-felt positive emotion. But when it does work, gratitude becomes a powerful mood booster and a step toward the 'upward spiral' to greater emotional well-being. The key is to persevere while remaining relaxed about the outcome. Accept that sometimes practising gratitude will connect to a positive emotion and sometimes it won't.

Once you get into the habit of gratitude, you often start to spot things during the day that will make it onto your gratitude list later. You can add to the benefits of gratitude by looking at what your involvement might have been in making the good thing happen. This builds confidence as you start to notice the link between your actions and the good things it results in later.

'Three Good Things' was included in Prof Martin Seligman's early studies on positive psychology interventions and was shown to lead to a lasting increase in happiness and decrease in depression, with the effects felt months later.[5] It can be used as a coaching or therapy technique to focus a client's attention on what is working well in their life. I use it at the start of a session to help the client get into a positive, resourceful frame of mind. It is also a good bedtime routine to establish with young children to nurture the development of a grateful disposition in them. By encouraging children to reflect on their good things, you are helping them to develop a mindset of appreciation of life rather than focus on what's missing. Opposite is a list showing some areas of gratitude to get you started (make these personal and specific to you).

Psychologist David Pollay suggests thinking of gratitude as having four foundation stones.[6]

✦ Firstly, gratitude reminds you of the **key people** in your life who love and support you. This is significant because we know that having good relationships is a characteristic of happy people.

✦ Secondly, gratitude acts as a reminder of your **strengths**, the natural talents that help you to move forward and reach goals.

✦ Thirdly, gratitude for the things that you have already **achieved** reminds you of the road travelled so far.

✦ Finally, gratitude acts as a reminder of the **wonders of the world** such as the miracles of nature, like how mighty oaks can grow from tiny acorns.

It is tricky to force yourself into feeling grateful, which is why Robert Emmons recommends trying instead to cultivate a disposition of gratefulness, which is the tendency to feel gratitude frequently.[7] People with this mindset see life as a gift and notice the many blessings they receive. The clue is often in the language they use, employing words such as grateful, thankful, blessed and gifts. Experiment with using the language of gratitude to turn it into a habit.

GRATITUDE LIST

✔ Health

✔ Home

✔ Neighbourhood

✔ Family

✔ Friends

✔ People who support you

✔ Achievements

✔ Work

✔ Living in a safe country

✔ A temperate climate

✔ Pets

The Gratitude Journal

The idea behind the gratitude journal is to record a list of all the positives in your life. Think of it as an extended version of 'Three Good Things', a 'good news' journal, which is the antithesis of the doleful Dear Diary that many of us used to record our deepest fears as angst-ridden teenagers. The act of writing it in a journal helps you to process your thoughts and raises awareness of the good that does exist in your life, as well as your role in making it happen.

Mette Dencker, a Member of Parliament in Denmark, frequently named as the world's happiest nation, keeps a gratitude journal. 'When I go to bed, I write ten things that I'm grateful for. It's a great way to go through the day from start to end and think of all the good things that have happened. And I add a "because" to everything that I'm grateful for. That way I don't just appreciate what happened, I also go through why I'm grateful for each little thing.' Mette's daily practice feeds the upward spiral: 'The more grateful I am, the more things happen every day that make me even more grateful.'

Doing this practice less frequently, maybe once a week, can prevent it from becoming a chore. I do it on a Sunday evening, which is a good time to reflect back on the previous week and look ahead to the week coming. Choose a notebook you'll treasure and use a nice pen. Or take the tech route and use a gratitude app on your smartphone.

The gratitude journal is a mighty tool in developing a mindset of abundance. As we look back over our lives it is all too easy to recall losses, missed opportunities, relationship breakdowns and the plethora of pain that accumulates as we get older. The gratitude journal contains the evidence of all the good times, which you may otherwise forget. As I look back over my old journals, it's like getting a second taste of them. Another way of doing gratitude is to write all your good things on post-it notes and put them in a large pot, such as an old-fashioned sweet jar. Ideally, start on 1 January and open it up on New Year's Eve to celebrate all the positives in the year that has been.

A cynic would say that it is all very well feeling thankful when things are working out in your life, but what about when you have suffered a misfortune and are feeling down? Well, actually, gratitude sometimes requires a degree of contrast or deprivation in order to experience its full effects. So while noone would ever recommend a loss of some kind, it does mean that when a need is filled after a period of absence, you will have a sweeter experience of gratitude. You appreciate the rain after months of drought or new work after a job loss. Losing something of value in one area of life can lead to a greater appreciation in other areas. The stressed-out executive, who quits to 'spend more time with the family' may experience a fresh appreciation of their loved ones, which might not have been the case had they continued with the high-pressure life.

Stressful events can also act as a prompt for gratitude. When I had surgery I remember experiencing waves of heart-felt thankfulness. Facing the reality of mortality renews appreciation for life itself; there was gratitude to the friends who supported me and appreciation of the surgeon's skill and the nurses' care. Imagining the bad stuff that might have happened but didn't can spark a torrent of appreciation – a near miss in the car, getting an 'all-clear' diagnosis or keeping your job during a period of redundancies. People who engage in this positive counterfactual thinking tend to be happier than those who don't.[8] There is also evidence to suggest that those who are able to feel gratitude in the wake of a trauma, such as being thankful that you still have your health or sanity, are better equipped to cope positively with the distress. They may even experience post-traumatic growth as a result of finding some silver lining in the trauma such as greater personal strength (*see* post-traumatic growth, p153).

Thank-you therapy

A really good way of amplifying the benefits of gratitude is to express it to others, thanking people for what they have done for you. Gratitude nurtures relationships and is beneficial for both the giver and receiver with goodwill bouncing back and forth between you. A friend of mine, Clive, carried out his own experiment with gratitude while we were training in positive psychology. He wrote handwritten notes on luxury stationery to express gratitude for good service he'd received – thanking the people at a go-kart business who'd laid on a birthday party to which his son was invited and to the owners of a newly-opened deli. On both occasions Clive was specific in his appreciation and each time he received a note back thanking him for his thanks! Gratitude helps us feel more connected and acts as a social lubricant helping us to bond with others and not take people for granted. It goes hand-in-hand with acts of kindness in increasing trust in society and adding to the tonnage of happiness in the world. In one of the early studies of positive psychology interventions, participants were asked to write a letter of thanks to someone who had been a positive influence on them in the past, such as a teacher or relative. They then hand-delivered the letter, reading it out loud in a 'gratitude visit'. The results were an immediate and substantial boost to the participants' happiness.[9]

A NOTE OF THANKS

Dear..............,

I'm writing to thank you for the support you have given me in the past when ....

....

....

Writing a thank-you note creates an event to savour (*see* next chapter). Use stationery you find appealing, listen to music that puts you in the mood to reminisce, and treat yourself to something tasty as you write your letter. If you want to practise thank-you therapy on a larger scale you could host a gratitude party for everyone you'd like to thank. The research suggests that you get better results from performing acts of kindness across a shorter time span so try expressing your thanks in a single day or event to maximize the positive emotions.

Gratitude is now making its way into the fields of education and business. When I do groupwork I often begin by asking the participants to check in with their 'Three Good Things' as a way of keeping track on the progress they've made since the previous session. In the intervention that I ran with vulnerable young people misusing alcohol, gratitude came out as the most successful strategy in raising happiness and the one that was still most often practised after the end of the programme. This holds true not only for young people living on the margins of society but also for the most privileged. Wellington College, one of the UK's best-known independent schools, runs a well-being programme. I asked one of their teachers which of the practices they used had had the most positive impact on the students? Gratitude ranked alongside meditation in top position.

Appreciative Inquiry

The art of appreciation is making its way into the workplace in the form of 'Appreciative Inquiry' or AI, a process of organizational development based on the idea that every individual or team has something positive to offer. The first step in AI is to appreciate the existing skills and strengths across the workforce, asking questions such as: 'What is good about what you're currently doing?'[10] The process of change works with the assets in the organization rather than the deficiencies. You can use a similar approach with the people in your life; what do you appreciate in your loved ones, friends, colleagues, neighbours or community? What's working well? What is there to appreciate?

Gratitude across time

Gratitude is a positive emotion associated with the past (appreciating what has been gained) but it can also help to generate good feelings about the future. Having the evidence of what went well before helps develop confidence in the possibility of things going well in the future, too. Gratitude is the glass half full looking back whereas optimism is the glass half full looking forward. Gratitude, can, therefore, stimulate optimism, which makes it doubly valuable because optimism (*see* p109) is one of the major thinking tools in tackling depression.

The one to read
The Little Book of Gratitude by Robert Emmons

CHAPTER 5

Savouring the Moment

+ **What is it?** Savouring is the ability to tune into, appreciate and enhance the positive experiences in your life.[1]
+ **In other words:** Extracting maximum enjoyment
+ **Try this for:** Positive emotions, happiness; building enjoyment of the present; as an aid to mindfulness and flow.
+ **If you like this, try also:** The Attitude of Gratitude (Chapter 4) and Meditation (Chapter 6).

~

*It is a lovely sunny morning in August as I begin to write this chapter. I make my favourite breakfast – juicy blackberries, now in season, with peaches and apricots. On top I add soya yogurt and oats, which **taste good** and I know will **do me good**. I take breakfast into the garden,* *luxuriating* *in the warmth of the sun on my back and* *feeling thankful* *that I am able to start the working day this way. Every so often I take a break to harvest some cherries,* *marvelling* *at how one small tree can produce so much fruit. I feel* *grateful* *to the previous owners, who planted the tree. This year I've been baking with fresh cherries rather than preserving them as I usually do. Cherry pie and cherry and almond tart so far, and* *what's really good* *is that it's eco-friendly with zero food miles! I'm* *relishing* *the idea of making a cherry clafoutis, a French dessert that I first had when I lived in France as a student. One summer, I was helping out on a film shoot in Paris. Feeling shy, I'd wander off at lunchtime but, one day, the director sent someone to find me to join the rest of the crew in the bistro. They were wondering where I was. I felt* *cherished* *and* *basked* *in the warmth of their friendship. That was when I had the cherry clafoutis. Back in the garden I* *appreciate* *the blogger who has posted a recipe for cherry clafoutis online.*

~

In this short (but true) story are many of the features of savouring, one of the processes that helps us to cultivate positive emotions. Savouring is about appreciating the good. You'll be familiar with the usual meaning of savouring – to actively enjoy the taste of something. In positive psychology savouring is the capacity to appreciate and enhance positive experiences in life. It's about getting the full flavour of a positive experience, deepening the enjoyment on offer. By *sharing* this story, I'm also using one of the strategies that intensifies the savouring.

You can savour just about anything as well as mouth-watering delicacies. Here's a random list to get you started:

+ The beauty of nature – the landscape, oceans, seasons, sunrise and sunset, the night sky.
+ Time spent with loved ones, the warmth and support of friendships, the delight and innocence of young children, the wisdom of elders, the skills of colleagues, the kindness of strangers.
+ A great book, a good film, a brilliant game, an uplifting concert, an inspiring piece of art or well-executed design.
+ Simple pleasures such as a hug, a laugh, fresh bedlinen or a nice warm bath.
+ Personal achievements, celebrations, special occasions such as birthdays, graduation, weddings, anniversaries.

The aim of savouring is to accentuate the positive, with an intention of generating positive emotions. Like gratitude, savouring helps overcome the negativity bias, the brain's tendency to pay more attention to the negative than the positive. They work well together – gratitude is about noticing what's good, while savouring is about making the most of it so that you squeeze all the juice out of a positive experience. Savouring has much in common with flow (*see* Chapter 2) and mindfulness (*see*

Chapter 6) but they are not identical. While savouring focuses on the positive, flow puts the focus on the activity – full immersion with a loss of self-consciousness – while mindfulness puts the focus on the present with deliberate non-judgmental attention to what is happening.

Depression is almost a form of reverse savouring, where your awareness of the negative deepens, 'savouring' the bleakness, the ashes and the utter greyness of life. This is what happened somewhat comically for a client of mine, when she headed to the local park for her first deliberate attempt at savouring. Determined to savour all the lovely aromas of nature she breathed in deeply, but it was the smell of doggy doo-doo that assailed her senses!

Once you get the hang of it, savouring is one of the most effective positive psychology techniques you can practise. It was by learning how to savour the positive that I was able to screen out more of the negative and begin the recovery from depression. The five senses play a key role in the process of savouring and here you can play to your personal preferences.

+ Some people favour the **visual** and will get a lot out of feasting their eyes on something beautiful, such as a work of art or a wonder of nature.
+ Others are more **auditory** and relish the sound of great music, singing in a choir, birdsong or even the rainfall on a window when tucked up snug and warm indoors.
+ Those who have **smell** as one of their stronger senses have all the marvellous fragrances of nature,

from flowers to herbs, as well as the many scented products. When I smell eau de cologne I am instantly transported back to the happy times spent with my grandmother.

✦ Those who like **touch** might enjoy a hug or luxuriate in a massage or a nice warm bath.

✦ And of course there are the many wonderful **tastes** of food. Some of my favourite flavours include the spicy sweetness of satay, a creamy Brie, a ripe mango, tart raspberries and the crisp elegance of a glass of Sauvignon Blanc. I could go on!

What do you like to savour? Begin a list using the senses as prompts – note your favourite sights, sounds, fragrances and things you like to touch and taste. Below are some ideas to which you can add.

~

*Savour the **sight** of ... nature, dawn and sunset, the changing colours of the seasons, flowers, tall trees, pebbles on the beach, a beautiful work of art, the many guises of your favourite colour in both nature and products, the kaleidoscope of colours in mosaics and stained glass, houses with pastel-painted fronts.*

*Savour the **sound** of ... music, your favourite radio show, the sea, rainfall, birdsong, bells, laughter, a language that charms the ear.*

*Savour the **smell** of ... flowers, grass, perfumes and body lotions, suntan oil, scented candles, essential oils, baking, a barbecue.*

*Savour the **feel** of ... walking barefoot on grass, a massage, a pet's fur, cool marble tiles, the sun on your skin, a furry hot water bottle.*

*Savour the **taste** of ... your favourite foods.*

Over to you ...

....

....

....

....

....

....

....

....

....

....

....

....

....

....

How to savour

Savouring is something that you do rather than something that just happens. It requires your active engagement but the pay-off is worth it. The more you get into the habit of savouring, the more frequently you will experience positive emotions and grow your capacity for happiness. There are four steps that can help you get into savouring, with one caveat – relax and enjoy the process. Don't get hung up on whether you've got it right or not.

- Slow down and stretch out the experience
- Engage your full attention
- Use all your senses
- Reflect on the source of the enjoyment

Slowing down is important. Happiness and health grow as we slow down the pace of life. This goes against the grain of the frantic pace at which we live in the 21st century with its fast food, instant messaging, speed dating, etc., but it is vital to take your time when you want to savour the positive.

In workshops I bring out a bowl of exquisite fruit and chocolate truffles to practise with. Eating a strawberry at half the speed and with twice the attention makes for an infinitely more pleasurable experience. Using the senses helps – notice a strawberry's bright red colour, its light fragrance, how the texture changes as you bite into it, and the sweet taste.

The Slow Movement is the very embodiment of savouring, a cultural shift toward slowing down the pace of life in order to fully appreciate its joys.[2] Best known of all is Slow Food, which is about taking the time to really appreciate the food you eat as well as the pleasures of dining with friends, eating locally-sourced food (like cherries from my tree) and slow cooking – think of how a casserole's flavour improves with time.[3]

The Slow Movement's many branches provide clues as to how we can apply savouring to various areas of life.

Slow Travel: Savouring the journey by engaging with local culture and people, rather than rushing to tick off sights from your to-do list.

Slow Parenting: Letting kids have the time to be kids and enjoy their play rather than pressurizing them into early achievement at school or elsewhere.

Slow Cities: Urban spaces that seek to improve the quality of life of their citizens with lots of green spaces and traffic-free zones for pedestrians.

Slow Sex: Slowing down to intensify the pleasure of physical intimacy. I'll leave the rest to your imagination!

Hunt the good stuff

One of the steps involves reflecting on the source of pleasure. So if you're savouring a strawberry you might be thinking back to summer holidays, remembering eating strawberries and cream, watching the tennis, making jam, etc. Good questions to aid reflection include *'What is good about this?'* Or, if you're savouring a memory, *'What was good about this?'* Or *'What do I value here?'* A note of caution, though. I used to have a dreadful habit of asking myself 'but am I happy?' right in the middle of an enjoyable experience, which would instantly puncture the happiness and make it evaporate. There is a fine line between reflection and overthinking something. It's all about engaging with the experience and being fully present to it rather than stopping to assess it. This is where the senses have such a useful role to play in helping you to stay connected to the moment.

The risk of compromising your pleasure is shown by an experiment in which three groups were asked to listen to a recording of some classical music.[4] The first group simply listened to the music, the second were told to try to make themselves as happy as possible while listening. The third group were asked to adjust a movable measurement scale to indicate their moment-by-moment level of happiness as they listened to the music. Which group do you think got the most enjoyment?

It was the first group, who simply listened to the music. The second and third groups found their experience was adversely affected. When you focus too much on examining positive feelings, as opposed to just experiencing them, it can disrupt the pleasure and short-circuit the savouring.

Type of savouring	**BASKING**
What?	The warm enjoyment of a reflected accomplishment, when something that you have done is met with recognition, admiration or congratulations
Focus	Self
Experience	Reflection
Examples	Basking in praise, triumph, glory, the glow of a job well done
Results in	Pride (in its positive sense of recognizing your success)

Type of savouring	**LUXURIATING**
What?	Delighting in physical pleasures, enjoying bodily sensations
Focus	Self
Experience	Absorbed in something physical
Examples	Luxuriating in a nice warm bath, sunbathing, sexual intimacy, a massage, a gourmet meal, fine wine, walking barefoot on grass, pampering, doing nothing
Results in	Physical pleasure

Type of Savouring	**MARVELLING**
What?	Transcending the self to experience a sense of wonder at something awe-inspiring or to commune with something bigger than the self
Focus	Outside the self
Experience	Absorbed in the sheer grandeur of something vast and/or impressive
Examples	Marvelling at nature, the universe, the divine, a higher power, a person, science, technology, music, an achievement
Results in	Awe, wonder

Type of Savouring	**THANKSGIVING**
What?	Reflecting on your good fortune and being flooded with feelings of gratitude toward the agent of that positivity
Focus	Outside the self
Experience	Reflection
Examples	Becoming aware of a good thing in your life, winning against the odds; near misses such as accidents, recovery from life-threatening illness
Results in	Gratitude

Based on *Savouring* by Bryant and Veroff

Savouring processes

At the forefront of research are American psychologists Fred Bryant and Joseph Veroff, whose book *Savoring*[5] describes a number of strategies to encourage, prolong and intensify enjoyment of a positive experience.

Bryant and Veroff have boiled savouring down into four distinct varieties: basking, luxuriating, marvelling and thanksgiving (gratitude), which we explored in the previous chapters. Cherishing is another form of savouring, within relationships (*see* Chapter 9).

Because depression puts you behind the starting line when it comes to savouring, give yourself permission to bask, marvel and luxuriate, and let go of any anxiety or moral judgment over the desirability of doing so. As with everything it is a case of balance, and any type of savouring can have a shadow side if taken to excess. Too much basking might transform a sense of natural pride into arrogance, for example, and luxuriating could become overly self-indulgent.

Savouring for success

Savouring is, as the old saying goes, about slowing down to smell the roses. There are some pre-requisites to make it work. Firstly, you have to be in a frame of mind where you are able to put aside concerns and worries and, secondly, you need to be able to focus fully on the experience. Mindfulness techniques can help with both these aspects (*see* p99). Multi-tasking, on the other hand, does not help – you need to focus attention on just one thing at a time. This also helps with managing stress. Having been a multi-tasking queen until I crashed into a mid-life depression, I now regularly stroll around my local park and stop to smell the fragrance of the flowers, squeeze a stalk of lavender or appreciate the trees with their changing foliage. This break in the middle of a busy day has many benefits – it calms me and helps to clarify my thinking so that I am in a better frame of mind to return to my work. It's a win-win situation as taking breaks to savour things means I generally end up achieving more.

We know that savouring produces positive emotions and positive emotions broaden our thinking processes, enabling us to be more innovative and flexible. So here is a justification to take a break to slow down and savour – it helps us to think better!

Sharing the pleasure is one of the most powerful ways of savouring; this draws your attention to the array of delights on offer. Being in the company of others who are having a good time can help you be more open to enjoying yourself and they may point out some aspect of the pleasure you've not yet noticed. Sharing an experience helps to bond people and strengthens a relationship. It's not just participating either; the act of watching loved ones enjoying themselves is in itself pleasurable.

Sharing the experience is a particularly good approach for extroverts. If you are more introverted, you might prefer practices that you can do alone, such as absorbing yourself in a riveting book. Boost this immersion by consciously tuning into certain stimuli (the beautiful, scented flowers growing by the roadside) while ignoring others (the cars). You can also take mental snapshots to form a memory of the positive experience. I did this on my first trip to Sydney, taking a ferry into the harbour with the Opera House on one side and the Harbour Bridge on the other. I truly immersed myself, drinking in every detail – marvelling at the feat of engineering that is the Harbour Bridge, appreciating the beauty of the shell-like curves of the Opera House and reflecting on its status as an icon of the Southern Hemisphere.

When something good happens, another form of savouring it is to adopt expressive, exuberant behaviour, in which you speed up rather than slow down – whoop with joy, punch the air, bounce up and down, dance around. Give yourself a big pat on the back when you have performed well, reflect on a job well done and think of how others will be pleased. It may feel counter-intuitive to give yourself such overt praise and can, of course, be inappropriate in certain situations, but there is evidence to suggest that outwardly expressing positive feelings can enhance them, so it is worth having a go.

The frequency of positive emotion counts more for happiness than its intensity,[6] which means you're better off going for quantity of savouring rather than the quality of the experience. Capitalize on the opportunities that come your way as you go about your day. A lot of savouring is about reacting, but here are some ideas for proactive savouring, beginning with this simple exercise.

EVERYDAY SAVOURING

Once a day, take the time to slow down and enjoy something that you would usually hurry through, such as eating a meal, walking somewhere or taking a shower. Afterwards write down what you did, how you did it differently and how it felt compared to when you usually rush through it.

Based on Positive Psychotherapy[7]

The savouring schedule

✦ Plan your week to include a daily savouring session lasting at least 20 minutes.

✦ Choose activities that you can look forward to and include variety in your schedule.

✦ At the end of each session plan the next day's activity so you can relish the idea of it coming up.

✦ Every evening look back on that day's experience to rekindle the good feelings involved.

✦ At the end of the week, take some time to look back over all seven sessions and see if this re-ignites any of the positive emotions you felt. Compare to how you would normally feel.

✦ A similar idea is to make yourself a playlist (*see* p52) and choose something to savour from it each day.

Based on Bryant and Veroff

PICTURE THIS!

The growth in digital photography and smartphones has made it so much easier to take a snapshot whenever you find yourself in an experience that you'd like to treasure. Make sure you stay engaged with the experience rather than thinking about camera angles. Review the photos from time to time to savour the memories. You could post the pictures on a social media site to share the experience. Or start a project to take one picture every day, or on the first day of each month, to savour a whole year.

Modern technology is a great aid to savouring. I find a smartphone invaluable for capturing the moment and creating a library of positive memories, and I use the pictures as screensavers. The images remind me of the joys of the moment, which I might otherwise forget. Research shows that the memories we recall tend to match the mood we're in, so a negative mood prompts a negative memory. As depression leaves you with very little sense of the good times, digital snaps can provide you with a potent reminder of their existence.

Savouring across time

Savouring is about appreciating something that is happening in the present moment but you can also savour across time. You might reminisce about a past pleasure or relish the anticipation of future pleasures.

Savouring the past

Positive reminiscence is the savouring of good memories from the past. This can have a beneficial impact in the present, boosting happiness levels and reducing emotional distress. It's a coping strategy that helps people feel better, escape from their problems and gain insight and perspective to tackle current difficulties. Positive reminiscence can remind you of your strengths and abilities, and help you build confidence. The risk comes when positive reminiscence is used solely as a means of escape, leading to negative comparisons with the present and living in the past.

Positive reminiscence can be aided with the use of a prompt or a prop. This could mean creating a picture in your mind linked to the memory, running through the events in glorious detail, sharing the story of it with someone, looking at memorabilia or playing music associated with the memory.

The senses play a role here too, as the 19th-century French novelist Marcel Proust famously demonstrated in *Remembrance of Things Past*, in which the lead character eats a *madeleine*, a small tea cake, which transports him away from the dreariness and depression of the present to an experience of all-powerful joy. Similarly, a quote from another French author, Albert Camus, shows how he was able to draw on positive memories to sustain him, *'In the midst of winter, I found there was inside me an invincible summer'*.

Positive reminiscence can be especially beneficial for older people, for whom the past may provide a richer source of satisfaction than the present. Doing a 'life review', for example, can generate a sense of personal achievement. The evidence shows that positive reminiscence can promote well-being and enhance self-esteem in later life. I interviewed many older people in my earlier work as a social historian and found that those who actively reminisced were among the happiest and liveliest of interviewees. This is confirmed by research on time perspectives.[8] People who are heavily oriented toward a 'past positive' perspective, associated with a warm, pleasurable view of their past, enjoy higher self-esteem and happiness.

Reminiscence is used as a therapeutic process that brings together families, generations and communities. I've seen it facilitate friendships among older people who have shared memories of a particular time. Here is an activity to get you started on positive reminiscence.[9]

SAVOURING A HAPPY MEMORY

Compile a list of some of your happiest memories. It could be a golden period in your life, maybe your time at college, one of your best holidays, falling in love, the birth of a child, a work success, climbing a mountain, etc.

Next, choose one of those positive memories to reflect on. Relax, make sure you're sitting or lying down comfortably, take a deep breath, close your eyes and summon the memory to mind. Imagine the event in all its glory, allowing impressions to float freely across your consciousness. Run through the details. Notice who was present, the expressions on their faces, what was said, the environment you were in, the colours, the temperature, the ambience and the feelings you had at the time. Reflect on what was good about the experience.

This can be a co-coaching exercise, where one person savours a memory while the other one acts as the coach, encouraging reflection by asking, 'What was good about it?' Another possibility, if you like writing, is to do it as a journaling activity where you tell the story of the experience in rich, vivid detail.

Based on Bryant, Smart and King[9]

Savouring the future

Anticipating future pleasures may seem impossible to do in depression, however it offers benefits to those who succeed. Having something to look forward to creates hope, positive feelings about the future and the motivation to make it happen. It gives you a chink of light in the darkness of depression. It is very easy to believe that there is nothing to look forward to, so this is where it helps to write a list of good things coming up, regardless of whether they excite you or not. This is about compiling evidence of positive events in the future.

In periods of depression I write lists in my journal of things to look forward to. It could be something like getting together with a friend or summer being just around the corner. If you find there is absolutely nothing, then that is your cue to sort something out – plan a get-together, a walk or a trip of some kind.

Give yourself permission to fantasize about what is coming up. Visualization is a tool used a lot in positive psychology to set goals and develop optimism. Savouring something as yet unknown comes with pros and cons. It can be a disadvantage in the sense that you may lack reference points to imagine how it will turn out, but it can also be an advantage because you are free to indulge in your fantasy without restriction. You can draw on the past as a reference point. So, if you enjoyed the last time you went to stay with a friend, savour what was good about the experience and then project those same feelings forward to the next time you do it. Relish the anticipation.

There are two questions that help with savouring the future. Ask yourself:

✦ What is good about this?
✦ What am I looking forward to?

Many people find that the future is the most challenging of all the time dimensions to savour, regardless of whether or not they are experiencing depression. Give it a try and see what happens.

Savouring is one of the foundations in positive psychology and it is well worth mastering the art of it. By doing so you're opening yourself up to a wider and deeper experience of the pleasurable and positive.

The one to read
Savoring by Fred B. Bryant and Joseph Veroff

CHAPTER 6

Meditation:
The Mindful Approach

- ✦ **What is it?** Mindfulness is a form of meditation that is about paying attention in a particular way; on purpose, in the present moment, and non-judgmentally.
- ✦ **In other words:** Training the mind to be aware of what's happening on the inside and outside, being present, observing without becoming attached.
- ✦ **Try this for:** Calming the mind, recovery from depression and anxiety, positive emotions.
- ✦ **If you like this, try also:** Savouring (Chapter 5) and Vitality (Chapter 10).

Meditation has been a spiritual practice in the East for thousands of years. In the West, it was often used as a means to relaxation but now scientists are discovering that it has many benefits for mental health, in particular for sufferers of depression and anxiety. I first became convinced of the merits of meditation for low mood when I discovered a neuroscience study that showed that regular practice of mindfulness meditation activates the area of the brain associated with positive emotions – the left prefrontal cortex.[1] Remarkably, it seems that regular meditation practice can *grow* your capacity for happiness.

Lean to the left

Prof Richard Davidson, from the University of Wisconsin, is a neuroscientist particularly known for his studies on the effects of meditation on the brain. His research suggests a left–right division in the brain's set points for mood. When people are emotionally distressed – anxious, depressed and angry – the most active sites in the brain are around the amygdalae (almond-shaped centres of fear) and the right prefrontal cortex. When people are in a good mood, those sites are quiet. Instead there is heightened activity in the left prefrontal cortex.

Davidson discovered that a quick way of working out someone's typical mood range is to assess the levels of activity in these left and right prefrontal areas. The more the activity tilts to the right, the more unhappy a person tends to be, while the more activity there is on the left-hand side the happier they are. Davidson has scanned many brains, including those of Buddhist monks (who make a lifelong practice of meditation), and found that regular meditators have much higher activation on the left-hand side.[2]

This news is like sweet music to the ear of anyone who suffers from chronic low moods. Here is a way to develop that 'muscle' for joy, love, contentment and other positive emotions. I was inspired to try the experiment for myself, practising mindfulness meditation daily over eight weeks – and yes, it did work. I did experience more positive emotions, though I might not have recognized them if I hadn't been keeping a mood diary as they were more subtle than the peaks of bliss and ecstasy. Instead I felt calm, relaxed and less anxious.

It was a joyful relief after many years of stress and marked a turning point in my life. I went from believing that I might be incapable of happiness to realizing that I was, in fact, consumed by stress. Through meditation I was able to calm down a perpetually busy mind and could tune into life's joys more easily. My ability to savour increased too. I was at the home of a friend one evening when her cat came in from outdoors. I leant over to stroke Louis and found myself going into raptures over his 'chilled fur'!

Meditation involves two main practices – concentration and mindfulness, which are frequently combined. Concentration is about focusing attention in a sustained fashion on an object and, when the attention wanders, bringing it back. It could be a candle flame, your breath or a mantra that you repeat. It's in the nature of the mind to wander, so this about gently redirecting your attention back to the object.

BENEFITS OF MEDITATION

MORE

- ✔ Positive emotions
- ✔ Happiness
- ✔ Resilience
- ✔ Ability to handle stress
- ✔ Ability to relax
- ✔ Satisfaction with life
- ✔ Energy
- ✔ Openness
- ✔ Self-esteem
- ✔ Self-acceptance
- ✔ Self-actualization
- ✔ Creativity
- ✔ Enthusiasm
- ✔ Learning ability
- ✔ Trust
- ✔ Self-control
- ✔ Empathy
- ✔ Spirituality

LESS

- ✘ Depression
- ✘ Stress
- ✘ Anxiety
- ✘ Loneliness
- ✘ Hostility
- ✘ Neuroticism
- ✘ Pain
- ✘ Relationship issues
- ✘ Negative body image

Mindfulness meditation

Mindfulness is somewhat different. There is no particular focus involved; it is instead a process of paying attention to your ongoing experience, whatever it may be at that moment. So, if you have lower back pain you pay attention to that – not by trying to concentrate on it, but simply by noticing it and letting it be. Mindfulness means 'awareness' or 'bare attention'. It is about being fully awake to the here and now, living in the present, connected to the flow of every experience, and conscious of how body and mind affect each other. The opposite is mindlessness, a feeling of being on autopilot, disconnected, obsessed with the past or fearing the future. Mindlessness is a way of wandering through life reacting automatically to people and situations, succumbing to habits such as stuffing yourself with food without noticing what you're eating or wasting endless hours in front of the TV. Mindless habits like these often steer us off-course on our path to greater well-being.

Mindfulness meditation is now recognized as a treatment for depression and one that helps prevent people from relapsing. It is particularly helpful in dealing with the effects of stress, which strengthens negative networks in the brain and weakens positive ones, leading to burnout. It can reverse the symptoms of the chronic stress response. By staying in the present you avoid being overly-oriented to past stressors, which can trigger depression, or toward future stresses, which can set off anxiety. Mindfulness helps you respond to stressful situations in a more reflective style rather than reacting automatically to try and deflect the pain.

MINDFULNESS ...

- Helps us to experience the world directly without the endless commentary of our thoughts.

- Helps us to experience thoughts as mental events that come and go like clouds and as ideas that aren't necessarily true.

- Helps us to live in the present rather than dwelling on the past or worrying about the future.

- Helps us to become more self-aware and stops us coasting on 'autopilot'.

- Helps to interrupt the cycle of mental events that cause us to spiral into depression.

- Stops us from trying to force life to be a certain way and helps us to become more accepting of what is.

The Buddhist monk and author Thích Nhat Hanh describes this as avoiding the urge to chase away unpleasant feelings and choosing instead the more effective path of returning your attention to your breathing, observing the bad feeling quietly and giving it a name, such as sorrow or anger, so you can recognize and identify it more clearly.[3] Rather than engaging with the negative feeling or thought and trying to suppress it, mindfulness encourages us to observe and be more accepting of it. Attempting to avoid or alter the intensity or frequency of an unwanted mental experience can – paradoxically – keep it going and set off the familiar triggers. By accepting rather than resisting, we may find that unpleasant feelings go away by themselves. What you resist persists! Equally, when we give up trying to force pleasant feelings, they are freer to emerge on their own.

My own practice tells me the truth of this. By taking regular breaks to meditate and letting go of always being in control, I found that there was rarely a cost but that plenty of good, unexpected things occurred, which convinced me of the value of taking time out to do it.

Mindfulness meditation helps with two of the major features of depression – emotional reactivity and rumination. This is a way of gaining awareness of our emotional and thought patterns, which enables us to step back more and manage our emotions better so that we stop the knee-jerk reactions to stress triggers. When adversity strikes many of us react as though on autopilot, interpreting events as threatening and uncontrollable. When we are able to pause we gain mastery over how we *respond* rather than *react* to stress. Meditation training allows us some distance, it gives us more of a bird's-eye view on a situation and therefore more flexibility in the way we respond. Mindfulness can also help to interrupt the loop of rumination, where we get stuck in a thinking track that pulls us down, winds us up or stresses us out.

Neuroscience has confirmed the many benefits of mindfulness meditation, including its effectiveness in reducing anxiety and negative emotions.[4] It can be a relief to learn that people who undergo mindfulness training show an increase in activation of the area of the brain associated with positive emotions, which is generally less active in those who are depressed. What this means, in effect, is that the more you practise mindfulness the more you develop your capacity for positive emotions and happiness. The best-known programmes for depression are **Mindfulness-Based Stress Reduction (MBSR)** and **Mindfulness-Based Cognitive Therapy (MBCT)**. Others such as Acceptance and Commitment Therapy (ACT) and Dialectical Behaviour Therapy (DBT) also have elements of mindfulness.

Mindfulness-Based Stress Reduction (MBSR)

Jon Kabat-Zinn is the pioneer who developed Mindfulness-Based Stress Reduction (MBSR)[5] at the University of Massachusetts Medical Center in the late 1970s. The MBSR programme is an eight-session mix of meditations and yoga practices and has been used with tens of thousands of hospital patients with a variety of psychological and physical illnesses such as generalized anxiety disorder, chronic pain, cancer, fibromyalgia and multiple sclerosis. MBSR has a track record of reducing anxiety and depression[6] and has now extended beyond clinical settings into the wider community. A quick web search will help you find a programme near you.

Mindfulness-Based Cognitive Therapy (MBCT)

Mindfulness-Based Cognitive Therapy (MBCT)[7] brings together Mindfulness-Based Stress Reduction (MBSR) with Cognitive-Behavioural Therapy (CBT). Mindfulness differs from CBT in that it encourages people to accept their thoughts without identifying with them rather than to challenge them. People are told not to aim for a specific result but simply to practise mindfulness and see what happens.

MBCT was developed in the 1990s to train people who suffer recurrent depressive episodes in techniques that disengage from automatic negative thinking, which can precipitate depression in susceptible individuals. Rumination, in which the mind repeatedly reruns negative thoughts, is a key factor in people relapsing into depression and even minor increases in sadness can reactivate the neural pathways of depressive thinking. Mindfulness is an alternative way of experiencing negative emotions that can prevent those emotions leading to depression. MBCT teaches people how to shift their mental gears to avoid being dragged into the downward spiral.

The expert practitioners behind MBSR and MBCT have collaborated on a book, *The Mindful Way through Depression*,[8] which includes a CD of meditations narrated by Jon Kabat-Zinn. This would be a good way to sample these mindfulness programmes.

FIRST STEPS TO MINDFULNESS

1. Whenever possible, just do one thing at a time.

2. Pay full attention to what it is that you are doing.

3. When your mind wanders from this, gently bring it back.

Kabat-Zinn suggests that bringing even a tiny bit of awareness to a single moment can help to break the chain of events that leads to chronic unhappiness. Begin by choosing some routine activity that you do everyday and resolve to do it mindfully, bringing a moment-by-moment awareness to the task. Applying mindfulness to the washing up is a classic way of starting to practise. So you might notice the sensations as you put your hands into the warm water in the sink, how the temperature changes as you adjust the taps, the aroma of the washing-up liquid, the rhythm of washing and stacking plates, the twinkling of newly-washed cutlery, the contrast as the crockery goes from dirty to clean and the feeling of completion when the task is done. You can also apply this mindful approach to other domestic tasks, as well as eating, brushing teeth, showering or driving. Directly sensing the messages that the body is giving us serves to lessen the persistent mental chatter going on in our heads.

Mindfulness Practices

Below are some of the best-known mindfulness practices for you to try.

MINDFUL BREATHING

1. Find a comfortable position, either sitting or lying down. If you are sitting down, make sure your back is straight and allow your shoulders to drop.

2. Close your eyes.

3. Focus your attention on your breathing. Notice what it feels like in your body to slowly breathe in and out. Make sure you are breathing correctly – as you breathe in, your belly goes out.

4. Now pay attention to your belly; feel it rise and expand every time you breathe in and feel it sink as you breathe out.

5. Immerse yourself fully in the complete experience of your breathing.

6. Whenever you notice your mind wandering away from your breath, simply notice what it was that took your attention away and then return to your breathing in the present moment.

7. Continue for ten minutes, or more if you prefer.

MINDFULNESS ON THE MOVE

Some people prefer a more active form of meditation to the sitting practice of mindful breathing where we withdraw our attention from the outside world. Walking mindfully is a form of meditation on the move with a greater awareness of what's going on outside – the environment, the elements, the people – while maintaining a focus on the experience of walking. Walking is also a good way of increasing awareness of our physical bodies. For your first attempt find an open space such as a park where you can walk uninterrupted for 15–20 minutes without having to deal with any traffic. You might want to try it barefoot as well.

1. As you stand on the spot notice how your weight connects to the ground through your feet. Notice the sensation of your feet in contact with the ground, your shoes, socks, etc. Let your arms hang naturally as you begin to walk.

2. Walk normally but slow down the pace to increase awareness. Keep your attention on the soles of your feet. Note how you raise and drop each foot, the contact with the ground followed by the release and how your body shifts with each step.

3. Take your attention up through your body as you walk. Consciously relax each part.

→

4. Notice what emotions happen to be present and what is going on in your mind. When thoughts unrelated to walking come up, just let them fade and return your attention to experiencing the walking.

5. Try to keep a balance between your awareness of your outer and inner worlds.

Once you've got the hang of this, then every routine journey becomes an opportunity for mindfulness on the move.

THE RAISIN EXERCISE

This is an exercise that many therapists use to introduce their clients to the detail involved in attending to something mindfully. You don't have to use raisins but choose a food that is small and easy to handle – grapes or blueberries are good alternatives.

1. Spend a minute looking at the raisin, noticing its colour and texture. Then take a moment to notice its scent.

2. Next, put the raisin in your mouth but don't chew it. Move it around your mouth and feel the texture of it with your tongue.

→

3. Then, take one small bite out of the raisin. Notice the difference between the taste and texture on the inside and outside.

4. Once you've noticed everything there is to notice, try eating the raisin slowly, aware of everything you taste and feel.

You may have noticed that mindfulness has a lot in common with savouring. Indeed it does, but they are cousins rather than twins. Emotions may or may not be involved in mindfulness but they are definitely the target of savouring.

THE BODY SCAN MEDITATION

This is a mindfulness exercise that helps us get a sense, in the moment, of what's going on in our internal landscape with our physical and emotional sensations. The body scan is a good way to ground or centre yourself and can help you regroup after an upsetting situation. I recommend lying down and taking your time to check in with each body part slowly and in detail, but you can also do it standing up. Get hold of a guided meditation to talk you through, or alternatively put on some relaxing music to accompany your meditation.

→

1. Lie down, make sure you are comfortable, close your eyes and begin by getting in touch with your breathing. Notice where your body makes contact with the bed or the floor. Take a few deep breaths to ground yourself.

2. Start with either the toes of one foot or at the crown of the head and slowly scan your attention up or down, depending on your starting point. The idea is simply to feel deeply into each part – bone, muscle, organs, blood flow, etc – and notice what is present in the body. Notice what is tense, relaxed, hot, cold, numb, tingling. Whatever you notice is present in the body in that moment is what you pay attention to.

3. Adopt an attitude of gentle curiosity to investigate the quality of the sensations that you find. The intention is simply to notice what is, not to feel different or relax, although this may be a happy consequence.

4. Move along in sequence, so if you start with the toes of one leg, move slowly upward. Notice what is happening in your feet, lower legs, calves, knees, thighs, pelvic region, lower back, stomach, mid-back, chest, shoulders, arms, hands, neck, face and head. Spend a few minutes in each area, deepening awareness into whatever is present.

→

5. When the mind wanders, acknowledge it, noticing the thoughts and emotions, remain mindful and gently return your attention to your breath and the body part you were scanning.

6. Don't worry about getting it right, if it is 'working' or not. The scan is a way to reconnect with the body on a deeper level and recognize the links between bodily sensations, thoughts and emotions.

Loving-Kindness Meditation

Besides mindfulness, Loving-Kindness Meditation (LKM) has also come under the scrutiny of psychologists for its benefits to mental health. This meditation is one of Buddhism's most ancient and is about cultivating states of warmth, love and kindness so that we become more compassionate all-round and treat ourselves and others with kindness. In Buddhist theory happiness comes from empathizing with others and seeing their suffering and well-being as being equally important as our own. By recognizing that one of our needs is to help others meet their needs, we shed a layer of self-centredness and find a path toward happiness.

Prof Barbara Fredrickson, the psychologist renowned for her work on positive emotions, has investigated this ancient practice by conducting experiments where individuals deliberately direct loving, kind feelings toward themselves, then to loved ones, then acquaintances, strangers and, finally, all sentient beings.[9] The results of her studies show that practising LKM increases a wide range of emotions, including love, joy, gratitude, contentment, hope, pride, amusement and awe. The rise in positive emotions is matched by a decline in symptoms of depression and an improved sense of satisfaction with life. Other benefits include an increase in self-acceptance, positive relationships and physical health.

Such is the efficacy of LKM that Fredrickson has suggested it as a remedy for one of positive psychology's biggest challenges – the 'hedonic treadmill'. This is where we adapt to our source of happiness and begin to take it for granted so that, over time, it has less effect. We even become accustomed to the ultimate joy of being in love. LKM produces such a variety and abundance of positive emotions that it helps to keep things fresh and may be a way to outpace the 'hedonic treadmill'.

LOVING-KINDNESS MEDITATION

May you be safe

May you be happy

May you be healthy

May you be peaceful and live with ease.

The How To of Loving-Kindness Meditation (*Metta Bhavana*)

LKM is the first in a series of meditations in Buddhism that produce four qualities of love starting with friendliness (*metta*), then compassion (*karuna*), then appreciative joy (*mudita*) and finally equanimity (*upekkha*). Approach this meditation with an open heart toward yourself and others. This is something you can do at home – there are plenty of LKM recordings online, or try your nearest Buddhist centre to learn the practice.[10]

- Begin with directing a loving acceptance toward yourself. You may experience resistance initially to the idea of this but the practice of this meditation is designed to overcome self-doubt and negativity.
- Send loving-kindness toward yourself and then systematically to each of the four types of people listed below.

1. Someone you respect such as a spiritual teacher
2. Someone you love dearly and unconditionally – a close family member or a friend
3. A neutral person – somebody you know, but have no special feelings toward, such as an acquaintance or someone who serves you in a shop
4. A hostile person – someone you are currently having difficulty with

The intention here is to break down the barriers between you and these four types of people with a parallel effect of also breaking down divisions within your own mind, the source of much of the conflict we experience. Try sending loving-kindness to different people, as some won't fit easily into the categories above, but keep to the prescribed order. If you find it hard to get started, maybe think of someone that's easy to love or perhaps a pet. Here are some hints to help develop feelings of loving-kindness.

Visualization – bring to mind a picture of the person the feeling is directed at and imagine them smiling at you or simply being joyous.

Reflection – reflect on the positive qualities of the person and their acts of kindness. Reflect, too, on your own positive qualities and make positive affirmations about yourself.

Sound – repeat a mantra or phrase to yourself such as 'loving-kindness'.

Buddhists suggest that Loving-Kindness Meditation be treated as more than a formal sitting practice removed from everyday life. They recommend taking it out into the world and directing an open-hearted, friendly attitude to everyone you come across. French-born Buddhist monk Matthieu Ricard recommends once an hour spending as little as ten seconds sending out loving-kindness to wish someone well. This practice is not only beneficial for our own mental health but helps to nurture our relationships, more of which in Chapter 9.

Meditation has transitioned from being a spiritual practice into a secular practice, with proven benefits for well-being. Mindfulness and loving-kindness meditations are two major contributions of the East into the positive psychology field. I can heartily recommend both of them. What I liked about this approach is that I didn't have to think too hard, which is challenging anyway in depression. The commitment was to do the practice. However, the net result was so favourable that I felt as though my brain had been rewired for happiness. If you think you might prefer a more cognitive approach then turn now to the next chapter, on optimism.

The one to read
The Mindful Way through Depression by Mark Williams, John Teasdale, Zindel Segal and Jon Kabat-Zinn.

CHAPTER 7

Learning Optimism: Psychological Self-defence

+ **What is it?** Expecting positive outcomes (dispositional optimism); how we explain the causes of events (optimistic explanatory style).
+ **In other words:** Seeing the glass as half-full.
+ **Try this for:** Challenging negative thinking and overcoming pessimism.
+ **If you like this, try also:** Positive Emotions (Chapter 3) and Resilience (Chapter 8).

One of the double acts of depression is the way that negative thinking and emotions reinforce each other, dragging us down. While mindfulness can help us disengage from negative thoughts, it is the practice of optimism that challenges the thinking patterns in depression. I was convinced for many years that I was a natural-born pessimist and even if I wasn't born that way, circumstances had certainly contrived to turn me into one. I expected that life would be hard and believed that the only way to succeed was to massively overwork and make multiple sacrifices. Not surprisingly, I was prone to episodes of depression. The turning point came one winter when I was on my way home from a ski trip in the Alps. It was snowing hard by the time I reached Geneva airport and all flights had been grounded. My mood turned as bleak as the sky. I was stuck at the airport just like I was stuck in life and nothing was ever going to change. I slumped into a seat, resigned to a long wait and reached into my luggage for something to read. I fished out *Learned Optimism* by Martin Seligman and found out that it was possible to learn how to do optimism even if you were born a pessimist. This was the revelation that gave me the confidence that life could change and ultimately put me on track for greater happiness.

Optimism and pessimism influence the way we think and feel when we encounter problems. Optimists expect positive outcomes even in difficult situations, whereas pessimists expect bad outcomes and this leads to negative emotions, such as anxiety, anger, sadness and despair.[1] One of the most uplifting findings from this area of research is that you can develop into a more optimistic thinker – in spite of the legacy of your genes, upbringing or experience of life. Things are more flexible than we once thought. Fast forward two decades and I'm now a practising optimist and testimony to its mood-enhancing benefits. I say 'practising' as it's something

I still do consciously as a form of psychological self-defence. And that's why optimism is worth the effort, because it acts as a shield that protects you from spiralling down into depression. I teach the techniques now to my clients and many times I've witnessed a palpable sense of relief when someone successfully defeats the monster of a pessimistic belief.

How pessimism leads to depression

In a nutshell, pessimism puts you on a fast-track to depression, while optimism protects you from it – optimistic people are more resilient in dealing with life's stresses and able to bounce back easier than pessimists. If you are pessimistic about the chances of something working out, you're less likely to put in the effort and more likely to give up when you hit an obstacle. This, of course, makes it even more likely that the bad thing you've been dreading will go on to happen. It becomes a self-fulfilling prophecy. This is the essence of what Martin Seligman calls 'learned helplessness'.[2] You have a pessimistic belief that 'whatever I do doesn't matter' – there is nothing you can do to change or control a difficult situation and so you give up, lose hope and become helpless. Depression lurks in the shadows. Pessimists are also more given to rumination – they brood on the causes and consequences of their suffering, going over it again and again, triggering the downward spiral, as we've seen in earlier chapters.

Over 30 years of studies have found that people with a pessimistic outlook are more vulnerable to depression and other health issues.

Optimism – self-defence for the mind

Optimism is a way of thinking that relieves the negativity generated by pessimism. Optimists see the glass as half full. They expect good things to happen and have a sense of confidence about life working out well for them. If you expect something to turn out well, you're more motivated to put in the effort to ensure this happens. And because you put in the effort, it *is* more likely to happen. There are many benefits for optimists. They enjoy greater psychological and physical well-being, cope better when things go wrong and experience less distress, depression and anxiety. Optimists have better immune systems, recover faster from surgery and also live longer. When bad news intrudes on their life, they don't go into denial as you might expect, but focus instead on finding a way to solve problems. That's why they adapt better to negative events. For example, they're more likely to go to the doctor to get symptoms checked out and then stick to health guidance. The optimism about optimism is fully justified, as it's associated with many of the good things in life:

✦ Happiness
✦ Positive mood

✦ Satisfaction with life
✦ Good health
✦ High performance
✦ Success

Are there any disadvantages to optimism?

So far it sounds like optimists have all the advantages, but there are a few drawbacks:

✦ Optimists sometimes lean toward an inaccurate perception of reality, which results in them becoming unrealistically confident.
✦ They can see themselves as low-risk for certain diseases and may underestimate the health risks – of smoking, for example.
✦ They may be inclined to take part in more high-risk activities such as speeding, drinking and driving, and casual sex.

Optimists can be vulnerable to stress when they choose to deny their negative emotions or persist in striving in situations over which they have little control. One potential threat to their well-being is having their rosy view of life shattered by a serious trauma or loss. For a pessimist this would merely confirm their beliefs, but for an optimist it could lead to a breakdown in their worldview and a loss of confidence in their ability to influence events in their lives. However, the evidence suggests that optimists may still be better equipped to rebuild their world. Pessimists are more likely to go into denial when there is a difficulty, whereas optimists tend to face up to it. Pessimists pay more attention to dealing with the difficult emotions generated by adversity, whereas optimists focus more on dealing with the problem itself.[3]

What about pessimism?

I'm sure some of you are thinking that pessimism is the safer option, it's more realistic and you're less likely to be disappointed when things don't work out. If you're usually a pessimist, however, you probably know all too well how depressing it can be. Pessimism is a way of thinking that focuses on the negative, emphasizes problems and anticipates things going wrong. Pessimists expect the worst to happen and, when it does, it confirms that they were right all along to think pessimistically, which, in turn, reinforces a pattern of negative thinking. Pessimistic explanatory style is a painful way to think. In this form of pessimism, when a negative event happens a pessimist will generally explain the cause of it as personal ('it's all my fault'), permanent ('it can't change') and pervasive ('it'll affect everything').

A positive in pessimism?

There is a form of pessimism that is more positive than most. If you are the type of person who is always prepared; who carries an umbrella in case it rains; who figures out all the alternative routes to get to your destination in case of transport problems or who rehearses endlessly for a presentation, then you are likely to be a 'defensive pessimist'.

Defensive pessimism is a coping strategy that is often used to manage anxiety. What defensive pessimists do is to prepare for the worst. Think of it as the embodiment of the Scouts' motto to '*Be Prepared*'. Defensive pessimists habitually set low expectations to help 'cushion' the potential blow of failure and spend time playing through various mental scenarios, paying special attention to all the possible things that might go wrong. They then prepare hard for the task ahead to avoid or minimize the chance of failure. And, generally, it pays off. If you recognize yourself in this, then take heart. Defensive pessimism seems to be a good strategy for those inclined to worry. It helps you to gain a feeling of control and to channel that anxiety into the effort to perform well. The compensation gained from this form of negative thinking is that it can lead to better performance, higher self-esteem, progress toward your goals and to the development of supportive friendships.[4]

Two different ways of thinking

So how can pessimists enable themselves to think more optimistically? Optimistic explanatory style is the form of optimism that you can learn. Optimists and pessimists tend to interpret the events that happen to them in three opposite ways.

EXPLANATORY STYLES

We explain events in three ways:

Me	**Not me**
Always	**Not always**
Everything	**Not everything**

PERSONAL ... PERMANENT ... PERVASIVE ...

It's not so much what happens that counts, as the way you explain it to yourself. This is what marks the difference between optimistic and pessimistic thinking. So let's look at how a pessimist thinks when a bad event happens to them. This is their explanatory style:

+ **It's me** (personal)
+ **It's always** (permanent)
+ **It's everywhere or everything** (pervasive)

Here's an example of how this works in practice for a pessimist. Let's say they were unsuccessful at a job interview, they might think:

+ It's all my fault that I failed. They didn't like **me** (personal).
+ It's **always** like this. I'll never get another job (permanent).
+ **Everything** in my life is ruined (pervasive).

You can hear how depressing it is to be giving yourself such messages – that the misfortune is all your fault (personal), it's forever (permanent) and will blight everything (pervasive). An optimist thinks in the opposite way to a pessimist. So when something bad happens, they think:

✦ **It's not me** (not personal)
✦ **It's not always** (not permanent)
✦ **It's not everywhere** (not pervasive)

If we apply optimistic explanatory style to the same scenario of being unsuccessful at a job interview, this is how it might sound:

✦ It's not about **me**, they must have found someone more experienced (not personal).
✦ It's not **always**, I've been successful in job interviews before, I'm sure I'll get something eventually (not permanent).
✦ This bad news isn't **everything**. Other parts of my life are going well right now (not pervasive).

By thinking like this an optimist is able to minimize the negative impact caused by a bad event.

Think like an optimist when things go wrong

If you're a pessimist, try experimenting next time something bad happens by thinking like an optimist – not me, not always, not everywhere – to see if it helps reduce the emotional pain. Use the following three steps to help you do this:

1. Expand your focus to think of all the other factors involved in the negative event. Rightly or wrongly, optimists have a tendency to blame external factors (others, circumstances) for things going wrong rather than themselves.* This helps to preserve their self-esteem.

2. Remind yourself that it may not be forever and how things pass. Look to evidence of how things change. We change, the seasons change, every cell in the body will change. This, too, will pass.

3. Look at the bigger picture. So you might have had a disappointment in this area of life, but what other parts are working better? Think of home, work, relationships, health, finances, leisure, studies, meaning in life.

*Although this is characteristic of how optimists think, you should still take responsibility for your life choices.

Think like an optimist when good things happen

Optimists and pessimists also think in opposite explanatory styles when they're explaining the causes of positive events to themselves. When a good thing happens to an optimist, they think:

✦ **It's me** (personal)
✦ **It's always** (permanent)
✦ **It's everywhere** (pervasive)

So if something good happens such as having a successful job interview, an optimist will think that it was down to them (personal) – their skills, experience and performance on the day; that this good fortune is here to stay (permanent) and that it will have a beneficial effect on other areas of life (pervasive). For a pessimist it's the other way around. They think:

✦ **It's not me** (not personal)
✦ **It's not always** (not permanent)
✦ **It's not everywhere** (not pervasive)

So, when the pessimist is surprised to get the job they went for, they believe that it was a fluke rather than anything to do with them (not personal), that the good fortune won't last (not permanent) and that it won't improve the rest of life (not pervasive).

	OPTIMIST SAYS	**PESSIMIST SAYS**
Positive Event	**Me**: It is all down to me.	**Not me**: It's a fluke! Nothing to do with me.
	Always: This is here to stay!	**Not always**: It's just a one-off. It won't last.
	Everywhere: This good fortune will spread.	**Not everywhere**: But everything else is bad.

Negative Event	**Not me**: It's nothing to do with me.	**Me**: It's all my fault.
	Not always: This too will pass.	**Always**: It's for ever.
	Not everywhere: It's only this small area of life, other things are going well.	**Everywhere**: It's going to affect everything in my life.

Tune into your automatic negative thoughts

To change the way you think involves consciously interrupting your automatic thinking. The first step is to tune into this internal dialogue – the critical voice in your head – and notice what automatic negative thoughts are playing on your internal radio station. You may begin to recognize the flavour of your pessimism. Are you someone who often thinks that it is all your fault when things go wrong and ignores the circumstances?

Or are you someone who thinks that when it goes downhill then that's the way it will stay. I once worked with a self-confessed 'recovering pessimist', who flew in from the USA to facilitate a training programme. As a very tall American, he was unused to the fixtures and fittings of the standard British hotel room. The showerhead was set too low for him and he grouchily resigned himself to having to crouch down to use it. On day three he noticed a lever and lo and behold – the showerhead shot up! This is typical of the mundane way in which the permanence of pessimism shows up – you make an automatic assumption that something is fixed and can't change. Another manifestation of pessimism is when you over-react to something going wrong, magnifying it into a calamity.

Learning optimism

In positive psychology the major tool used to challenge pessimistic explanatory style is the ABCDE, which Martin Seligman outlines in his classic book *Learned Optimism*.[5] This model is at the heart of the Penn Resilience Program (PRP), which has been found to significantly reduce the incidence of depression in schoolchildren, for whom it was first developed. The ABC of the ABCDE is the way we interpret the events that happen to us, while the three Ds stand for the methods used to challenge the pessimistic thinking. The E is the reward when successfully applying the preceding steps.

A = Adversity: 'A' stands for the adversity, the bare facts of the event.

B = Belief: 'B' is your belief or thought about the adversity. This is your 'heat-of-the-moment' interpretation of what happened.

C = Consequences: These are the consequences for your emotions and behaviour. They are driven by your 'B's – beliefs about the adversity.

D = Disputation, Distraction, Distancing: 'D' stands for the three methods you can use to deal with the pessimism.

E = Energize: 'E' is the energy you regain when a pessimistic belief is successfully defeated.

Seligman recommends getting to know your ABCs so that you begin to recognize how it is your belief about what happens that drives the consequences for your emotions and behaviour rather than the event itself. Carry a notebook in which you list the adversities that happen, and sit down later and separate out the A from the B and the C. Use the example in the chart below to guide you.

A (Adversity) – A friend hasn't responded to the invitation to my birthday party

B (Belief) – She doesn't care about me

C (Consequences: how you felt and what you did) – I felt angry, upset, and I deleted her from my contacts

A (Adversity) – ....

....

B (Belief) – ....

....

C (Consequences) – ....

....

The next part involves tackling the pessimistic thought – the B – using one of the three **Ds – Disputation, Distraction or Distancing. Disputation** is the main tool here. Imagine you're a barrister in court, arguing with the pessimistic belief. Ask yourself these questions:

✦ What is the evidence for this thought? For and against?
✦ Is there an alternative explanation for what happened?
✦ What are the implications of holding this thought?
✦ How useful is it to me? Does it work for or against me?

The most powerful way of disputing a pessimistic belief is to show how it might be inaccurate and to do this requires *evidence*. Because the mind is automatically seeking out evidence that confirms the pessimistic thought, it is likely to miss out on the evidence that contradicts the belief. So, in the example above, while you may believe your friend to be insensitive for not responding to your invitation, maybe you're missing out on other evidence – for example, that the friend might be away and may not have picked up your message.

By examining the evidence you may discover causes for the adversity that are neither personal, permanent nor pervasive. This can feel a little clunky in practice as you attempt to interrupt the automatic negative thoughts, but it is worth sticking with and persistence does make it easier. You may even become able to talk yourself down from the habit of catastrophizing, defaulting to the worst possible outcome of what might happen, which is often the case with pessimistic thoughts as they spiral out of control. So in the example you might go from *'my friend's not answered my invitation and she doesn't care'* to *'none of my friends care'* to *'I don't have any real friends'* and then to *'noone cares about me'*. All because one person hasn't responded to an invitation.

You can see how these pessimistic explanations create distress and drive the downward spiral into depression. I frequently help coaching clients identify the evidence that will interrupt their mental sprint to the worst possible outcome.

Another way of disputing the belief is to look for *alternative* explanations, which are kinder, non-personal and less damaging – for example that the friend might not have seen the invitation. Focus on causes which are changeable or specific, such as the fact that this is the only time it has happened.

Ask yourself what are the *implications* for holding that belief? Even if you still take a negative view over what has happened, you can still take steps to decatastrophize. Even if this friendship has been damaged, what are the implications for your other friendships? This particular relationship may be on the way out but it doesn't mean you've lost all of your relationships.

Finally, how *useful* is it to you to have this belief? Does it serve you in a positive way? For instance, is it helpful to imagine that all your friends have abandoned you? Unlikely. These forms of disputation will help to challenge the automatic flow of pessimistic thinking.

The other two Ds in the ABCDE model stand for **Distraction** and **Distancing**. Both of these practices can help manage the intensity of emotions generated by the negative events, so that you can regain your composure. Then when you get back on track you can turn your attention to the process of disputation. What do you do when you need a distraction to give you time to regroup? You might pick up the phone to chat to a friend or go and make a cup of tea. Distancing is similar to distraction; it's about putting some distance between you and the pessimistic thoughts so that they have less of an impact. This could mean removing yourself physically by going for a walk or using distance of time by choosing to focus on the situation tomorrow. Or externalizing it by imagining that the negative thoughts are being uttered by someone whose goal in life is to make you unhappy. What works for you when you need to gain some distance?

A reframe – finding an alternative

Reframing is a very useful skill to combat pessimism. It involves finding a positive in a negative situation. So, say you were planning a Sunday walk in the countryside, but as the day dawned it was raining hard and the walk was cancelled. You ask yourself: how can I get something positive out of this? You could reframe it as an opportunity to have a long lie-in or head somewhere for a nice Sunday lunch. So, you look for a positive to take some of the sting out of a negative situation.

I've taught this technique to young people and found that it works particularly well as a first step in developing optimistic thinking. I remember one teenager I worked with who was living in a hostel but threatened with eviction, which would have made him homeless. He was facing a very difficult situation but amazingly 'Sam'* still managed to reframe it. He said that if he were evicted, he'd be leaving a place he had little liking for and might be temporarily housed in a bed and breakfast where the breakfast was free! Sam was evicted but ended up living with his mother, so his reframe may have helped him indirectly on the path toward a more positive outcome.

Is it possible?

A simple yet powerful question which can open the door to optimism in the most negative of thinkers is to ask: 'Is it possible?' So even if Sam had been deeply pessimistic about his situation, was it possible – in theory – that he could end up in better accommodation? Yes, it was. Is it possible that someone can find new love after a loss? Yes, it is. Or a new job after redundancy? Yes. Even if you are a die-hard pessimist, logic will tell you that all these things are possible. Being able to imagine the possibility of future positive events is a step toward having the confidence in them happening. This question, which I use in coaching, can help strengthen the brain's ability to do optimism.

*name changed

The overthinking trap

Overthinking is a pattern of examining and re-examining negative emotions, thoughts and memories, which is more prevalent in women than men. The inner monologue involves rehashing the past or worrying about the future. It is easy to become overwhelmed with these distressing thoughts once the mind starts spinning and overthinkers are left in a state of constant anguish over their inability to stop it, becoming vulnerable to depression and anxiety. Here are some tips to manage worrying.

✦ Distract yourself.
✦ Write your fears down. Putting them on paper can take the heat out of them in your mind.
✦ Avoid the triggers that set off overthinking – specific places or situations.
✦ Take one small step a day toward solving the problem. Before you know it, things will have moved forward.

TIME TO WORRY

This is an exercise for those who worry too much, are overemotional and prone to anxiety, depression and anger. The aim is to stop kill-joy interruptions to your day and save them instead for a specific time. This is useful when you find yourself 'sweating the small stuff' or struggling with things you have little control over.

→

- As soon as you notice yourself fretting over something, postpone the worrying by promising yourself that you'll think about the problem later in the day during a designated 'worry time'.

- Set aside 15–30 minutes for your 'worry time'. Choose a time when you know you'll be calm and collected, for example after some relaxing or physical activity.

- If you notice gremlins surfacing outside the 'worry time', try to distract yourself with a mindful practice (see Chapter 6), or some other activity such as physical exercise.

Based on *Quality of Life Therapy*[6]

Looking on the bright side

We've looked at how optimism tools can be applied to combat the negativity of pessimistic thinking but, of course, you can also use optimism to generate positive feelings about the future. One daily practice, which takes inspiration from the 'Three Good Things' exercise that we met in Chapter 4, is to think of three positive things that you expect to happen tomorrow, then choose one of the three and allow yourself to savour the positives associated with it, writing down the good things that you think might happen.

LOOKING FORWARD TO TOMORROW

- Think of three positive things that you expect to happen tomorrow. Write them down.
- Choose one and anticipate the positive feelings you associate with it. Spend five minutes maintaining these positive feelings.
- Repeat the same exercise every day for the next week.

Based on Littman-Ovadia and Nir[7]

This process of counting and contemplation, which is a future-focused version of 'Three Good Things', has been found to reduce pessimism, negative emotions and emotional exhaustion.

Another scientifically-grounded practice is an exercise known as 'Best Possible Self'. Psychologist Prof Laura King discovered that writing about your best possible future self has great benefits for psychological and physical well-being, including an immediate boost in positive emotions, an increase in happiness weeks later and, over the longer-term, lower rates of illness.[8] This is an approach to creating an ideal vision of the future based on realistic goals rather than fantasy.

People are instructed to consider their most cherished goals in each area of life and visualize what it will be like achieving those goals. Writing about your 'best possible future self' generates optimism and an abundance of positive emotions, as well as the hope that fuels the drive to make these goals a reality.

If you're familiar with journaling, you may already have some idea why writing about your 'best possible self' works well. The act of writing down your vision helps you to gain insight about what's really important to you, your priorities in life, and what motivates you. Plus, it can generate ideas about how to reach those goals and navigate around any obstacles. In this version, from a study by psychologists Ken Sheldon and Sonja Lyubomirsky, people were invited to do the exercise as often as they felt like over the course of four weeks. So if you like journaling, then this exercise could be a good one for you.

YOUR BEST POSSIBLE SELF

Find a peaceful, comfortable place to sit where you won't be disturbed. Take 20–30 minutes to think about how you would like your life to be in the future – one, five or ten years from now. Visualize a future in which everything has worked out for the best. You have worked hard and succeeded at accomplishing all of your life goals. Think of this as the realization of your life dreams, and of your own best potentials.

Based on Sheldon and Lyubormirsky[9]

Prof Sonja Lyubomirsky, author of *The How of Happiness*, recommends this activity as a way of developing the 'optimism muscle'. Like any new habit, optimism takes practice, so do persist with it. Eventually, you'll begin to see the brighter side of life and this will be infused with a heart-felt positive emotion.

Hope for the best and prepare for the worst

As with everything in life, optimism is all about balance. Blind optimism can get you into as much trouble as die-hard pessimism. Martin Seligman recommends developing a 'flexible optimism'.

When to choose optimism

✦ When you're concerned about how you will feel – keeping your morale up or fighting off depression.
✦ When the situation will be protracted and your physical health is the concern.
✦ When it's about an achievement.
✦ When you want to lead or inspire others.

When to choose pessimism

The guideline is to ask yourself what is the cost of failure in any particular situation. If it is high – endangering life or relationships – then it might be wise to choose cautious pessimism. So, in the case of a drunken partygoer contemplating driving home, it is better to choose the pessimism and take a taxi. You'd prefer an airline pilot to check out that funny sound in the engine before take-off.

Another psychologist, Sandra Schneider, suggests a hybrid combining optimism and realism, which she calls 'realistic optimism'.[10] This is about hoping for and working toward the outcome you desire but tempered by a realistic outlook, so that you have an accurate view of the situation (rather than looking at it through rose-tinted spectacles) and you know how to proceed to achieve success. It is not about expecting that something will land in your lap without having put in the necessary effort.

A word to the wise on learning optimism

I don't want you to feel bad if you find it hard to cultivate optimism. The thing about automatic negative thinking is that it is just that – automatic. The pessimism habit is a tough one to shift. Change certainly *is* possible, although questions remain over how large or permanent a change can be realistically expected.[11] The benefits of optimism are such that every little bit of repetition counts. Be kind to yourself, keep going, don't judge your efforts and be grateful for every step forward. Even after 20 years I wouldn't claim to be a natural optimist, rather a practising optimist, but it is definitely worth it.

The one to read
Learned Optimism: How to Change Your Mind and Your Life by Martin Seligman

CHAPTER 8

Resilience: The Road to Recovery

+ **What is it?** The ability to control how we respond to negative situations in life and bounce back from adversity.
+ **Try this for:** Coping positively, moving forward after a setback.
+ **If you like this, try also:** Positive Emotions (Chapter 3), Learning Optimism (Chapter 7) and Vitality (Chapter 10).

Breakdown, loss, conflict, bereavement and ill health are a few of the adversities we may have to endure at some point in our lives. Life is full of challenges, stress and suffering – it's an inevitable part of the human condition. But whereas some people go under when faced with a crisis, others bounce back. This is because they are resilient and, like happiness, you can grow your resilience.

Your reservoir of resilience

So far we've looked at how positive psychology can raise your well-being, now we focus on how to recover your well-being after a setback, trauma or loss. In Chapter 1 I mentioned a metaphor for resilience that I use in coaching and groupwork. Think of your resilience as being like the water level in a reservoir. If you feed the reservoir with some of the many resilience ingredients like optimism and positive emotions (*see* the diagram for others), then your level of resilience will rise and you'll be better able to sail over the rocks of life's adversities rather than crashing into them.[1]

There are three major forms of resilience:

Resistance: Your ability to stand strong during adversity with your feet planted firmly on the ground.

Recovery: Your 'bouncebackability', like the tree that bends and sways in a storm.

Reconfiguration: The positive changes that will make you better able to cope with future challenges.

Resilience is one of the major areas of research in positive psychology, aiming to equip people to reach for a positive outcome in difficult circumstances. This focus shows how positive psychology tackles the negative by asking questions, such as what are the positive ways of coping with difficulty? What works to support your ability to bounce back? And is there anything positive to be gained from your negative experiences? In this chapter we'll look at what helps.

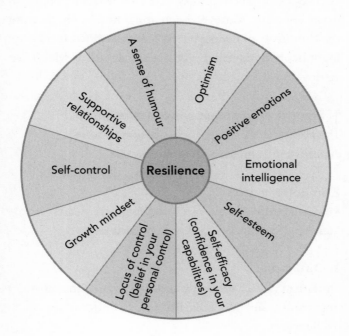

Ordinary magic

The good news about resilience is that it doesn't require extraordinary capabilities. Instead, it relies on basic skills such as being able to come up with a plan of action, and everyday ingredients such as friendships. Prof Ann

Masten, one of the experts in the field, calls it 'ordinary magic'.[2] As well as enabling us to bounce back from life's harshness, resilience also operates as a form of protection against the ill-effects of stress. Some resilience skills develop in childhood, but you can also pick them up as an adult. Karen Reivich and Andrew Shatté from the University of Pennsylvania have identified seven core ingredients in psychological resilience, all of which can be developed:[3]

1. Emotional awareness and regulation
The ability to identify which emotions you're experiencing and manage how you feel.

2. Impulse control
Resilient people don't rush into things, they can control their impulses and put up with uncertainty.

3. Optimism
Optimism (*see* Chapter 7) is arguably one of the most important resilience skills. Pessimism undermines resilience.

4. Causal analysis
Being able to think through why things happen and consider problems from different perspectives.

5. Empathy
Being able to understand the emotions of others.
This helps to deepen bonds and gain mutual support.

6. Self-efficacy

Having confidence in your ability to solve problems and using your strengths.

7. Reaching out

The ability to reach out to others, being willing to take calculated risks and being accepting when things don't work out.

Positive Coping

When a crisis hits, your first line of defence is your default coping style. People generally use one of three forms of coping – emotion-focused coping, problem-focused coping or avoidance coping.[4] It's worth getting to know which style is yours because there are advantages and disadvantages to each, as you can see in the chart overleaf.[5]

Emotion-focused coping is when your attention is on dealing with the emotional distress, rather than on resolving it. Not every crisis has a solution to it, of course, nor is it within our control – such as in the case of a bereavement – so finding a way to manage the emotional pain may be the sensible option. Emotion-focused coping includes talking things through with a confidante or counsellor, the emotional release of crying and leaning on friends and family for support.

When you can, attend to overwhelming emotions first and then when you feel calmer and have a clearer

Emotion-focused coping	Problem-focused coping
POSITIVE	**POSITIVE**
Processing emotions	Accepting responsibility
Talking things through	Developing a realistic action plan
Leaning on friends for support	Seeking accurate information
Crying – emotional discharge	Using optimism
Exercise and relaxation	
NEGATIVE	**NEGATIVE**
Seeking meaningless support	Procrastination
Taking the stress too seriously	Developing unrealistic plans
Alcohol and drug abuse	Not following through on strategies
Embarking on destructive relationships	Pessimism
Aggression	
Unproductive wishful thinking	

head, you'll be in a better position to find solutions. This is the essence of **problem-focused coping**, where your attention is on what steps you can take to resolve the issue. It's a more active form of coping, appropriate for adversities in which you can exercise some control, such as in the case of a business failure. By taking on the responsibility and coming up with a plan of action, you have a map to help you move forward. While it's important to deal with the emotions involved, eventually it will pay off to develop more of a problem-focused strategy, so that you can pick up the pieces and start over.

Avoidance-coping, is as the name suggests – about blocking out the crisis and engaging in distractions. Denying the existence of a problem sounds like an all-round negative, but in the short-term it can serve a purpose as a distraction that can help you regroup before tackling the issue. This depends on choosing a healthy distraction, such as social activities rather than something unhealthy, such as drowning your sorrows in drink. Over the long term, though, you are better off facing up to the issue and finding a way of managing it rather than turning a blind eye and risking things getting worse.

Take a moment now to identify your usual style of coping. Think back over the last crisis you faced. What did you do? Was your focus on dealing with the emotions, solving the problem or on distracting yourself from the pain? How might the other styles serve you?

✦ If your style is emotion-focused, try coming up with an action plan.

+ If your style is problem-focused, consider whether you might benefit from some emotional support to address your feelings.
+ And if your behaviour is avoidant, then take a deep breath and turn your attention to what's going on. What actions could you take to improve your situation?

The ABC of resilience

The Penn Resilience Program (PRP) is one of the best-known courses in resilience skills, developed by psychologists at the University of Pennsylvania.[6] Central to the PRP is the model of Adversity-Beliefs-Consequences (ABC) that we met in the previous chapter, which shows us how our beliefs about events impact our emotions and behaviour. Through this model people learn how to spot the errors in their thinking, evaluate the accuracy of their thoughts and challenge negative beliefs by coming up with alternative explanations. Here's a reminder:

+ When an *Adversity* happens ...
+ You have a *Belief* or thought associated with it, which is your interpretation of what happened. This *Belief* leads to ...
+ *Consequences* for your emotions and behaviour – how you felt in that moment and what you did, even if you did nothing.

The adversity is simply the fact of what happens. The same adversity could be a minor irritant to one person and a major calamity to another, because of the different beliefs they have in play. Resilience is about taking control of the parts that you can change. You may not have much control over the adversity, but you can influence your beliefs about it and that is the part we target. It's not so much what happens to us that counts but more the way we think about it, because it's our interpretation of what happens that drives the emotions and behaviour that follow on from it. So, to give you a simple example:

You're stuck in traffic (the *adversity*) and your *belief* might be that you're going to be late and lose your job (notice how these thoughts default to the worst possible outcome) and the *consequence* might be that you feel anxious (emotion) and take a risk attempting an illegal shortcut (behaviour).[7]

Getting familiar with your ABCs is a step along the road to developing resilience. The trouble is that these beliefs are so automatic that it can be hard to figure them out. You may find it easier to work backward because there are patterns in the connection between beliefs and consequences. So identify the consequences in the chart overleaf and then look to the left to find out what type of belief is triggering them.

An example of this working backward might be arriving home one evening to a note from the postman saying that he was unable to deliver a parcel and experiencing a fit of anger (the consequent emotion).

Working backward you might discover that the anger (the C) was generated by a belief (the B) that your Saturday would be ruined by having to go and collect the parcel. Use the chart opposite to fill in your own ABCs.

BELIEFS	← CONSEQUENCES
The belief is around...	**Emotions/behaviour**
Loss (I've lost something or someone)	Sadness/withdrawal
Danger (something bad is happening)	Anxiety/agitation
Trespass (I've been harmed)	Anger/aggression
Causing damage (I've done something wrong)	Guilt/reparations
Negative comparison (I don't measure up)	Embarrassment/ hiding away

Once you get into the habit of working out your ABCs, you may begin to notice your own patterns in thinking and emotions, and whether you tend more, for instance, toward sadness, anxiety or anger. It is these repetitive spirals of negative thoughts and emotions that can pull you down into depression.

Adversity	Belief	Consequences
(*What happened – the facts*)	(*Your interpretation*)	(*Emotions and behaviour*)
Bumped into neighbour's car	He's going to hate me!	I felt nervous (emotion) and avoided him (behaviour)

Tackling the negative beliefs that undermine resilience involves challenging how we think about adversity and adopting healthier ways of thinking. You've already seen most of these techniques in the chapter on optimism with the D of disputation (*see* p123). Dr Karen Reivich, lead instructor of the PRP and co-author of *The Resilience Factor*,[8] describes this as fostering *accurate* and *flexible* thinking. Accurate thinking is about weighing up the evidence that supports or challenges the beliefs that we hold. Flexible thinking is about being more malleable in the way we think, coming up with alternative and more optimistic ways of looking at the situation.

You may wonder why we don't just do this as a matter of course. What gets in the way is the perilous pair of the **confirmation bias** and the **negativity bias**.

The **confirmation bias** is the habit of seeing the evidence that supports our beliefs and ignoring evidence that doesn't. So we notice everything that fits with our worldview and miss all the clues that contradict it. If the negative belief is that you'll never get another job after being made redundant, you'll notice all the evidence that seems to support that, such as the economy being in a downturn. And you'll ignore the evidence that contradicts that belief, such as more people being in work than out of work even when the economy is in recession.

This is where the negativity bias teams up with the confirmation bias. The brain leads you to focus on what's wrong, such as sad stories of unemployment, and ignore the tales of success of those for whom redundancy marks the start of an exciting new chapter of life.

If you are depressed, your mind will be supplying you with evidence that confirms your depressing worldview, which can plunge you further into the downward spiral. Knowing that these biases exist is helpful, but that's only part of the story because the mind plays all kinds of tricks – mistaken assumptions and thinking errors that we are likely to fall into when stressed or depressed. These all hamper our ability to think flexibly. Taking a step back to observe our thoughts (mindfulness is great for this) will reveal how the brain operates, taking the negative on trust and mistrusting the positive.

Aaron Beck, one of the pioneers behind CBT, recognized that this 'distorted thinking' is linked to depression. Feeling low is driven largely by how we think about the world. By interrupting these automatic thoughts we can stop ourselves being sucked into the downward spiral. Below and on the following page is a list of some of the most common thinking errors. See if you recognize the ones you generally fall prey to. All these thinking errors are common, especially in depression, and give you a blinkered view.

THINKING ERRORS[9]

- **All-or-nothing thinking** This means thinking in absolute terms. 'Things are *always* going to be like this.' 'It *never* changes.' All-or-nothing thinking is a key player in depression. Challenge it directly: 'Always? Never? Is that really the case?'

➔

- **Mental filter** Focusing almost exclusively on one small element of an event, usually the most upsetting or negative part.

- **Magnifying and minimizing** Distorting reality by magnifying the negative in a situation (making a mountain out of a molehill) or minimizing the good.

- **Dismissing the positive** Continually running down or diminishing the positive aspects of a situation.

- **Jumping to conclusions** (usually negative). This can take the form of 'mind reading', making assumptions about what someone is thinking, or 'fortune telling' where you anticipate how things will turn out.

- **All about me** Thinking that you are the cause of all the misfortune that happens around you.

- **All about you** Blaming others and circumstances for adverse events and being blind to your own role.

- **Overgeneralization** Taking isolated examples and turning them into rules of how the world operates.

- **Emotional reasoning** Making decisions based on feelings rather than objective evidence.

- **'Should' statements** Inflexible patterns of thinking about how the world 'should' be, how others 'should' behave.

- **Labelling** Putting a negative label on people and events, for example labelling yourself as a loser.

Externalizing the negative belief by writing it down or talking it through with someone can help you see the mind's blindspots. You may not recognize that your beliefs are so negative, thinking that they are simply factual – for example, 'I've lost my job, I'll never get another one'. By writing it down, you can spot more easily that this is all-or-nothing thinking and jumping to conclusions. By examining the evidence you can separate the facts from the beliefs and begin to recognize your negative thinking patterns. Below is an example of someone cross-examining a negative belief. Have a go with one of your own.

Adversity: My relationship broke up.

Belief: I'll never be in a relationship again.

What's the evidence?

- I've been in a relationship for more years of adult life than I've been out of one.
- People form new relationships after divorce. I know X and Y (specific evidence) have gone on to have new relationships.
- You can form relationships at any age.

Adversity:

Belief:

What's the evidence?

....

....

....

I find the question, 'Is it possible?' (that we met in the last chapter, see p126) really useful here. So, is it possible that you could have a new relationship? Unless you live in a highly repressive society that bans relationships, the answer is most definitely yes!

Positive emotions fill your reservoir of resilience

Positive emotions play multiple roles in resilience. On a personal level they undo the effects of stress and help protect against depression, so that you find yourself able to bounce back more easily from negative experiences. On a national level, studies examining the aftermath of 9/11 in the USA, for example, show that the presence of positive emotions helped people find meaning in negative situations and accelerated their recovery from the trauma.[10]

Think of how a laugh can lift the mood even in the darkest of times. Humour generates positive emotions and this helps people to deal with adversity. By seeking out joyful experiences that put sunshine in the soul, you'll feel better and add to your resilience. Positive emotions loosen the grip of negativity on your mental outlook. Barbara Fredrickson, author of *Positivity*, places positive emotions at the heart of building resilience, putting the brakes on the slide into depression. Moments of feeling good enable you to regain your perspective and reverse the downward spiral.[11]

Having access to positive emotions marks the difference between people who experience stress reactions that dissipate fast and those for whom stress escalates and lasts for days. Positive emotions 'reset' the body back into the parasympathetic nervous system, returning the heart rate and blood pressure to normal. It's not that resilient people don't experience any negative emotions, it's just that they're better able to accommodate positive emotions alongside them. Refer back to the preceding chapters for practices that will help you fill that reservoir with positive emotions and raise your level of resilience.

For first-aid resilience, think physical

When we're in the middle of a crisis it can be hard to think straight, let alone think resilience. Physically, our bodies may be on full alert, in 'fight or flight' mode with the release of stress hormones such as cortisol and adrenaline. The amygdala (the part of the brain associated with stress, anxiety, fear and anger) is aroused. This is all counter-productive when a cool head is needed to deal with the adversity, which is why in the heat of the moment it often pays off to use your body as a first-aid kit. Doing something physical can flick the switch from the red alert of the sympathetic nervous system (which prepares us for 'fight or flight') to the calm of the parasympathetic nervous system (the rest-and-digest response), which helps us to relax and access a quieter place to think straight.

Resilience first-aid kit

+ Deep breathing
+ Any physical activity such as walking, jogging,
  dancing or swimming
+ Meditation
+ Yoga
+ Martial arts such as tai chi or qi gong

The body also plays a significant role in your underlying level of resilience. Think of how your ability to cope is compromised when you're tired, run-down, ill or not sleeping well. And how good sleep, decent nutrition, physical activity and an abundance of energy can help you to see things in a more positive light. Your physical well-being influences your resilience, so pay attention to the mind–body connection and remember how tending to your physical well-being will support your mental well-being.

Reaching out

Sometimes it's only when we hit rock bottom that we finally find a way out of depression. This can be the moment when we begin to reach out to others. So often we try to soldier on alone until we reach a point where nothing seems to be working. On a personal note it was only when I hit rock bottom that I noticed so much kindness and compassion in others, even strangers.

There will be people who want to help you out of the dark tunnel into the light, so pluck up the courage to reach out to them. You may be surprised by who turns out to be your angel of resilience. There is a fellowship in depression, of people who've been through the bleakness and understand what it's like. Support is not only to be found in those you know, there is also a community in self-help groups and online forums. Sharing your experience with others who have faced similar challenges can help you on the road to recovery.

Heroes of resilience

Other people can be a source of inspiration. Do you have a resilience hero? Someone who has overcome adversity? Who went from surviving to thriving? It could be someone you know personally – mine would be my grandmother in northern France who went through the Second World War and had to flee the farm she lived on during the Occupation. She was fired at and survived a piece of shrapnel lodging in her neck. Similarly, it could be a historical figure such as Nelson Mandela, who withstood 27 years of incarceration before becoming President of South Africa.

You can learn resilience from other people and the strategies they use. I have a friend who devours books about great feats of endurance whenever she's down. She finds it comforting and inspiring to read about people who've sailed around the world single-handedly or survived being kidnapped. It puts her misfortune into context to read about what others have had to suffer.

WHO IS YOUR RESILIENCE HERO?

1. What challenge did they face?

2. What strengths did they show to get through it?

3. What strategies did they use to survive?

4. What can you learn from their experience?

SSRIs: your personal resilience kit

A major source of resilience is your own past experience. I was introduced to the SSRI toolkit by my collaborator and friend, Dr Chris Johnstone, who has transitioned from being a medical doctor into a resilience specialist. He also has a history of depression. The term SSRIs normally refers to a group of anti-depressants, the Selective Serotonin Reuptake Inhibitors. Here they stand for **Strategies, Strengths, Resources and Insights** – all elements that can strengthen your resilience.

Think back to a difficult situation in the past that you got through in a way you are now satisfied with. What helped you through? What were the:

✦ **Strategies** you used? Practical things like asking for help, self-care, problem-solving approaches.

✦ **Strengths** you drew upon? Your inner resources such as courage and perseverance. Discover your strengths in Chapter 11.

✦ **Resources** you turned to? The external sources you relied on for guidance, inspiration or support. This could be friends, family, colleagues, mentors, professionals, support groups, online forums and organizations.

✦ **Insights** you found useful? Ideas, perspectives, philosophies and phrases that helped you through, like 'this too will pass' or 'whatever doesn't kill you makes you stronger'.

Based on Personal Resilience in an Hour by Dr Chris Johnstone
(www.udemy com.)

Beyond resilience: post-traumatic growth

It may be some consolation to learn that even in life-shattering adversities where things can never be the same again – the death of a loved one, a natural disaster, acts of terror or war, a terminal diagnosis or a life-changing injury or illness – there can still be positives. Not only do we have the capacity to bounce back from adversity, we can also grow through it. This is a phenomenon known as **post-traumatic growth** – positive changes that occur as a result of attempts to cope in the aftermath of traumatic life events.[12] This is not about denying the suffering or some kind of token compensation. Even in the worst of life events a hint of something positive can emerge. Enlightenment and growth can co-exist with trauma and despair. Here are some of the benefits reported by people who've experienced post-traumatic growth.[13] They gain:

✦ **A 'better self'**; feeling stronger – 'if I can get through this, I can get through anything'; more alive, authentic and open to what life has to offer; increased confidence, competence and independence; greater maturity and humanitarian instincts.

✦ **Stronger and closer relationships**; a greater appreciation of people, recognition of who your true friends are; increased love, empathy and compassion for others; greater sense of community and ability to relate to others, particularly with fellow trauma survivors.

✦ **Sense of meaning and purpose**; a fresh appreciation for the preciousness of life; a new and wiser philosophy on life; a spiritual awakening; a shift in priorities and new possibilities.

Post-traumatic growth is something that occurs naturally in events that shatter our view of the world. There are two ways in which people process trauma – **assimilation** and **accommodation**. Prof Stephen Joseph, author of *What Doesn't Kill Us*, has a brilliant metaphor for post-traumatic growth. Think of a beautiful vase that breaks into pieces. You can glue it back together again. It will look more or less the same, but have more cracks and be more fragile than it was before. This is what happens in assimilation. You try and integrate the trauma into your current worldview.

The other thing that you can do with a broken vase is to take the pieces and create something new out of it, maybe a piece of art such as a mosaic. So the vase becomes something new and more robust than its glued-together version. This is accommodation, where you modify your worldview to accommodate the reality of what's happened – and this is what can give rise to post-traumatic growth. Rather than focusing on re-building life exactly how it was before (assimilation), the aim is to build a life that will work within the new situation (accommodation). So, someone who is widowed is more likely to experience post-traumatic growth if they can adjust to being single. Accommodation involves accepting that random negative events can occur and the best you can do is to try and live with the here and now as much as possible.[14]

Writing about adversity

One way to reveal the hidden benefits in an adversity is to write about it. Putting distressing events into words is a form of catharsis, helping to get it off your chest, make sense of your experiences and find some kind of meaning in them.[15] It also helps to organize your thoughts so that you're more likely to come up with ideas about what to do next. James Pennebaker is the psychologist who has studied the therapeutic properties of writing about adversity. Although it can be upsetting as you relive what's happened, over the longer term even a short spell of writing for 15 minutes a day over four days has benefits for health, such as better immune-system functioning. One study carried out with a group of engineers who'd gone through redundancy found that the act of 'expressive writing' led to positives that included new offers of employment.

ADVERSITY JOURNALING

Want to give it a go? You may already be familiar with journaling, used as a personal development tool to process thoughts, gain insights and tap into creativity, such as in Julia Cameron's *The Artists' Way*. The idea here is to write in free-form, without stopping and without regard for the niceties of spelling, grammar, etc. Aim to keep going for 15 minutes at a time.

Over the next few days, I'd like you to write your very deepest thoughts and feelings about one of the most traumatic experiences of your life. In your writing, I'd like you to really let go and explore your emotions in depth. You may link your experience to your relationships with others. You may also want to link it to your past, your present or your future, or to who you have been, who you would like to be, or who you are now. You can write about the same general issues or experiences on all the days of writing or about different traumas each day.

Based on Pennebaker's The Expressive Writing Paradigm[16]

The ones to read

The Resilience Factor by Karen Reivich and Andrew Shatté

Seven Ways to Build Resilience by Chris Johnstone

CHAPTER 9

Positive Connections: Other People Matter

+ **What is it?** Relationships are the major source of happiness.
+ **Try this for:** Positive emotions, life satisfaction and well-being.
+ **If you like this, try also:** Gratitude (Chapter 4) and Savouring (Chapter 5).

'Other people matter' is how one of the founding positive psychologists, Chris Peterson, summed up the science of well-being.[1] We are social animals with a deep need to connect and belong. What the very happiest people have in common is that they are highly social and have strong relationships.[2] Depression creates a sense of disconnection, isolating us from other people who might support us and distract us from our pain. We are less likely to reach out because of a higher sensitivity to potential rejection. When we're on our own we're more likely to spiral downward. People who are alone or feel alone suffer more mental illness than those with strong networks. One of three fundamental needs for well-being is relatedness, the need to be understood, appreciated by, connected to, and the need to relate to and care for others. Even though depression makes us feel like being alone, the road to recovery is helped by doing the very opposite – nurturing our connection to others. Spending time with others is a natural anti-depressant that helps to lift the mood and reduce anxiety, emotional pain and stress. This chapter explores some of the ways we can build a sense of interpersonal well-being.

It's very easy in a consumer society to lose sight of the importance of relationships. Yet people who prioritize love over money are happier than those who put a premium on wealth. I remember one workshop in particular with a group of young people. During a discussion over what does and doesn't make us happy, I told them that money plays only a limited role in happiness and once your basic needs are covered, it ceases to have much effect on well-being. This was such a head-on clash with their beliefs that there was nearly a riot! For them money *was* the route to happiness. I then got them to do an exercise that involved savouring their happiest memories. Out came all these wonderful stories about falling in love, the births of babies and special times spent with loved ones. And that's when they got it – none of their cherished memories came with a price tag attached. The best things in life are free. The knowledge that happiness is more likely to be found in relationships than in retail therapy, gives you a strong clue as to where to invest your efforts. Prioritize the people in your life and cherish them.

Micro-moments of connection

In the 21st century the focus is much more on the 'me' rather than the 'we', whereas earlier generations put a greater emphasis on the needs of family and society. Martin Seligman links the epidemic in depression partly to this trend toward the self and individual satisfaction.[3] Maybe an antidote to that comes in the form of Barbara Fredrickson's research on love, the supreme positive emotion, which shows that it has multiple benefits for psychological and physical well-being.[4] Fredrickson's definition of love is 'positivity resonance', micro-moments of warmth and connection where you mirror the other person with a shared experience of positive emotion and behaviour, and a mutual impulse to care for one another. What I like about this is that it isn't the exclusive preserve of loved ones, you can have a micro-moment of connection with anyone, even a passing stranger. So try smiling at someone in the street.

The 5:1 positivity ratio for relationships

So what do relationships need to work well? Prof John Gottman at the University of Washington has discovered a positivity ratio, that is the ratio needed of positive emotional experiences (eg. being affectionate, kind or interested in each other) to negative ones (such as being hostile, critical, ignoring or hurting their feelings) for a relationship to flourish. The ratio is five positives to every one negative, which shows you how damaging negative experiences are to a relationship if you have to have five positive events to make up for it each time. Maybe a heart-felt apology (one), bottle of wine (two), cooking dinner (three), treats (four) and a foot massage (five)! Joking aside, Gottman has been able to predict with great accuracy which couples will stay together and which will break up based on the way they interact with each other.[5] The four most destructive behaviours within a relationship are defensiveness, stonewalling, criticism and contempt. Be warned!

Five good things

The negativity bias that makes us pay attention to what is wrong before we notice what is right also affects relationships. So you are more likely to tune into your loved ones' vices than you are their virtues. One way to counteract this bias and nurture your relationship is to actively remind yourself of someone's positive points, whether it's their kindness, loyalty, energy, sense of humour, work ethic, etc. This can also refer to the good things they've done. Gratitude smoothes the course of relationships and helps you appreciate the give and take in them. Think of five positives about your loved one to nudge you in the direction of the positivity ratio.

WHAT I LOVE ABOUT..

1. ....

2. ....

3. ....

4. ....

5. ....

Let's talk

The way you communicate can make or break a relationship. According to research carried out by Dr Shelly Gable at UCLA, there are four main styles in communication, ranging from active to passive and constructive to destructive, which are revealed by the way we respond to someone's good news.[6] Only one of these four ways of responding will nurture the relationship. Have a look at the example below to see if you can identify your habitual style and that of people in your life.

The good news	Typical response	Way of responding
I've got a new job!	'OK, that's nice.' (low-key)	PASSIVE and CONSTRUCTIVE Quiet, low energy support
I've got a new job!	'You know, my back's really playing me up today.'	PASSIVE and DESTRUCTIVE Ignoring the good news; changing the focus to yourself
I've got a new job!	'What about that extra stress you'll be taking on?'	ACTIVE and DESTRUCTIVE Quashing the good news
I've got a new job!	'That's really great! Is it the one you wanted? When do you start?'	ACTIVE and CONSTRUCTIVE Enthusiastic support, asking for details; leads to capitalizing

Based on Gable et al[7]

Active constructive responding is about responding to someone's good news with enthusiasm and energy rather than in other passive or destructive styles. By asking follow-up questions you can encourage the holder of the good news to come up with even more positives so they can capitalize on their positive event. It's the only form of responding that builds the connection and turns a good relationship into a better one. There are mutual gains – positive emotions, happiness, self-esteem and lower levels of loneliness. Interestingly, it is more important for the quality of the relationship to respond actively and constructively to the good news rather than provide a shoulder to lean on during bad times.

Social emotions

Emotions are contagious. They spread rapidly through groups, workplaces and communities. This holds true for both positive and negative emotions. A joyful mood can be infectious, passing from one person to another, but so can gloominess, bringing everyone down. Not only does your personal mood spiral up or down, so can the mood of the group around you. This is something to be aware of, especially if you are easily affected by other people's emotions. If you work or associate with people who are constantly moaning, the negativity will catch hold and spread. The brain has 'mirror neurons', which fire off in response to observing emotions in others.[8] What this means is that we pick up emotions from others and experience them directly. This is the reason why I choose to watch comedies on TV to catch the infectious humour and avoid the diet of depressing news.

Use this knowledge to spread delight rather than despair and keep people's spirits up. Point out the positives in any situation and try to overcome the collective negativity within groups. Here are some strategies to help you to manage the contagious nature of emotions.[9]

◆ Smiling is infectious. Smile and pass your good mood on.

◆ Other people matter, but avoid being drawn into other people's misery. You can be compassionate without joining in.

◆ Identify who are the 'radiators' and the 'drains' in your life. 'Drains' are the people who suck the energy out of you, whereas 'radiators' are people who make you feel warm on the inside.

◆ Create 'high-quality connections'.[10] These are built on mutual positive regard, trust and active engagement on both sides. Any point of contact is an opportunity for a high-quality connection. People feel engaged and open, which in turn increases energy and the likelihood of mutual support.

◆ Protect yourself from 'corrosive connections' – poor-quality connections that sap your energy. These are relationships based on distrust and a lack of regard. It can be hard to avoid corrosive connections if they come in the form of a boss. In such cases try not to take it too personally – it might simply reflect a lack of social skill in the other person.

The how-not-to of social comparisons

We humans have a toxic tendency to compare ourselves with others. Am I as successful? Happy? Attractive? Rich? Slim? This sense of competition runs deep as we judge our own opinions and aspirations by comparing ourselves with others, and this has a profound effect on our well-being.[11] Social comparisons affect us in all kinds of ways. For instance, studies have found that people would rather earn more money than their peers than earn more money overall. It's more important to be seen to be doing better.

If you're depressed then social comparisons are the ultimate feel-bad experience. You're more likely to feel wounded if you rate yourself to be lacking in some respect compared to someone else. This produces a noxious brew of negative emotions, such as envy, resentment, anxiety, sadness, anger or disgust, combined with low self-esteem and insecurity. Happy people are more likely to rise above self-punishing comparisons. They still make comparisons, but other people's triumphs have less of an effect on their personal well-being.

Compare down not up

Upward comparisons are those we make with people we perceive to be better off than ourselves. This can sometimes be a source of inspiration – when the other person's success is within your grasp. Then, it can fuel your motivation to achieve something similar. However, upward comparisons are frequently made to people who are not within reach, such as celebrities with their perfect-looking bodies and lifestyles. Upward comparisons can leave you feeling inadequate and down.

It's best to distract yourself from making unfavourable comparisons, but if you can't there is an alternative, which *does* help your well-being. That is to compare yourself downward to people who are less fortunate. It sounds like a rather dubious thing to do, but it does work. Comparing downward can help you appreciate what you have. It's a great antidote for the negative emotions generated by unfavourable upward comparisons. So, for example, I compare myself to people living in politically unsettled nations and this also has the added benefit of making me grateful that I live in a stable democracy.

Cherish the love

If relationships are the primary source of happiness, then to love is the ultimate practice to build well-being. Love is both a strength and a positive emotion in positive psychology. Moments of love are made up of a whole host of emotions, from joy and gratitude to serenity, hope, pride, amusement, inspiration and awe.[12] And the more moments you have, the more it raises your level of resilience. You begin to experience a sense of oneness, of community, which mitigates against the loneliness of depression. Love has many forms, from romantic love which matures into a more companionable love, to love for children, parents, other family and friends. And from the micro-moments of warmth to a wider love for people and the planet.

Cherishing love is a form of savouring (see Chapter 5) that can enhance the benefits of love. A way of doing that is by voicing your appreciation of the love you share. One long-term study of marriages shows that communicating the savouring of love to a spouse has a beneficial effect on the quality and resilience of the relationship. Bryant and Veroff offer tips on savouring a romantic partnership, which could equally be applied to deepening the bonds in other types of relationships.[13]

✦ Share interests and activities
✦ Pay close attention to the details of their life so that you appreciate their likes and dislikes
✦ Collaborate on a shared task
✦ Disclose things about yourself to promote intimacy

Sharing is not only good for relationships, it is one of the most reliable ways of raising the level of enjoyment on offer. Think of how you might share some of the practices in this book. Try making the 'Three Good Things' exercise (*see* p58) something you do with a friend or partner and build the feel-good factor between you.

Acts of kindness

The more you give the more you receive. Acts of kindness are win–win situations because not only do they help others to feel good but they help you to feel good, too. Altruism is just as beneficial for your psychological health as it is for your relationships. It may seem counter-intuitive when you're down but it really does work. Acts of kindness are about performing good deeds for others, whether it's offering support to someone in need or contributing your time to a worthy cause. Volunteering is often put forward as a remedy for the blues; it is a way of distracting yourself from your own problems and from rumination, one of the risk factors for depression.

Acts of kindness can be spontaneous or pre-planned. What works well, according to studies conducted by Sonja Lyubomirsky, is to inject variety into what you do to keep the kindnesses fresh and meaningful, and to concentrate the acts into a short period of time. This intensifies the power of kindness to boost mood.[14] But a word of warning – your good deed needs to originate in a genuine desire to help. If you feel coerced or obligated for whatever reason, the benefits of kindness are limited both for yourself and for the person receiving.[15] Your motivation needs to be intrinsic (kindness for its own sake) rather than extrinsic (kindness for a reward like greater happiness).

Performing random acts of kindness for complete strangers has evolved into a social movement, spreading joy and promoting global well-being. Another idea is to 'pay it forward', to do good deeds for others in recognition of having yourself been the lucky recipient of some unrelated kindness. If you're looking for inspiration, there are plenty of ideas on websites linked to this worldwide phenomenon.[16]

Forgiveness

If you're wondering what forgiveness is doing here, it's because forgiving others for the harm they caused is good for *your* personal well-being. Letting go is healing; it reduces depression, anger, anxiety and feelings of hostility, as well as helping your physical health by lowering stress and blood pressure.[17] I know it is easier said than done, but if you can view it as something you're doing for yourself rather than for the other person, you'll no longer be drinking from the toxic cup of negative emotions that a lack of forgiveness produces. Forgiveness is an antidote to resentment, anger and dark thoughts of vengeance. Even though the wish to retaliate may be strong, by giving in to the desire for revenge, you risk setting up a vicious cycle of escalating acts of harm.

Forgiveness is not the same as condoning, excusing, forgetting or denying the harm that has been done. Neither is it about being a doormat for someone's abusive behaviour or restoring the relationship with the other person. It's about responding to transgressions with mercy instead of vengeance. You don't have to have contact with the transgressor in order to forgive. You could write a letter of forgiveness without sending it. There exists a forgiveness movement that brings together victims with perpetrators to help the healing process.[18] In positive psychology forgiveness is recognized as a strength of character. By developing this strength, you can gain the virtue of temperance. Find out more about your strengths in Chapter 11.

Virtual friends

Recently I was home alone suffering with flu. I felt miserable and lonely. I posted an update on social media and within hours a stream of messages of support had arrived. It was like the sun coming out after a grey day. My mood lifted. I was alone but no longer lonely.

It's very easy to question whether these kinds of 'virtual friends' count as real friends. I prefer to think of social media as a way of opening yourself up to a new horizon of potential interaction and to view it as an addition to, rather than as a substitute for, socializing. Social media can give you a great sense of connectedness as long as it's not entirely at the expense of real-life connections. Through social media I am able to stay connected to friends in different parts of the world, to keep up with events in their lives, to make connections with people who have the same interests and to be part of a global community in my field.[19]

The downside is that people tend to display the better side of their lives on social media, which can trigger unfavourable social comparisons. You won't be surprised to hear that there is a limit to the number of 'friends' with whom you can maintain a meaningful relationship. What you may not know is that the number stands at around 150, according to evolutionary anthropologist Robin Dunbar.[20] This is the maximum number of social contacts that you can sustain in your personal network and still have some kind of quality within the relationship.

Appreciate your weak ties

It's natural and normal to value our close relationships above others, but there is also something to appreciate in our wider networks. Weak ties are those people we don't know so well, acquaintances who exist more on the periphery of our lives. You might think that many of your social media connections are weak ties, of little meaningful value compared to the strong ties in your life. However, in certain circumstances weak ties can be more beneficial.[21] The theory goes something like this: whereas our strong ties tend to move in the same circles as we do, weak ties move in different networks, so they provide a bridge into new circles of influence, resources and even jobs. So a network of social media friends, for example, can open up all kinds of new possibilities. This is the strength of weak ties and a reason to value those connections.

Married, single, other ...

I'm aware that a lot of this chapter reads as if couples win hands down in the happiness stakes and that single people fare badly. While it is true that getting married is one of the few things that can increase your set point for happiness, it is not as straightforward as it seems. For starters, the initial boost in well-being does tend to wear off eventually, although overall happiness levels are higher for the wed than the unwed. It is, however, the quality of the relationship that counts; being in a bad marriage is worse for your well-being than being single or divorced. Co-habiting couples also do well in terms of their happiness, although not quite matching the advantages of being in a good marriage. So, a secure, stable, successful marriage tops the league in terms of the benefits for well-being.

Single and divorced people are, according to studies, lower on happiness than their married or co-habiting counterparts. One of the reasons for this is because of the lack of readily available psychological support. After a rotten day at work, sharing your woes over a glass of wine helps to alleviate the stress and this is more difficult if you're living on your own. The answer for those not in a close, personal relationship is to build supportive networks around you. I've lived both the life of a singleton and the attached. The support I give and receive from my female friends is just as valuable as that gained from a partner. The difference is that you have to work that bit harder to develop those networks rather than having support on tap from a partner.

Our faithful friends

When it comes to getting over the black dog of depression, your pet may also have a role to play. There are many health benefits from being around animals. I have friends who attribute their recovery from depression to getting a dog. Here's what they say:

'Having a dog made me feel better because I had a dependent; the dog needs you to take it out and feed it. The dog gives you love and you have something to love in return. Dogs are upbeat, enthusiastic and when your dog is wagging its tail looking forward to the next thing, you can't help but be taken somewhere else in your mood.'

'I can honestly say that getting my dog was a significant part of healing for me, after my father died. I had lost interest in the world, gained lots of weight, lost confidence and stopped socializing. Getting Sabbi ensured I had to walk her outside each day, which had a twofold benefit: it connected me to nature, which was very nourishing and it got me exercising again, so I gradually started to lose the weight and gain a desire to interact with the world around me again.'

'What I realized was that getting a dog helped me not to fall back into depression. I had to look after something. It's the responsibility that made the difference. I've got to look after somebody else and so I have to look after myself.'

'It was kindly pointed out to me that my lurcher, Bob, is in fact my longest male relationship, currently running at ten years! Not only is he loyal, dependable and trustworthy, he is kind and loves me 100 percent unconditionally. Of course he helps with my well-being!'

With social isolation on the rise, dogs are great for making a connection – my friends can barely get around the park without half a dozen conversations with fellow dog-walkers. Owning a dog is social, it distracts you from rumination and develops your fitness thanks to all those walks. It can even lead to a romance – I know a couple who met through their pets and are still together 20 years later!

✦ Having a dog protects against depression
✦ It reduces stress and anxiety
✦ Dog walkers are healthier than non-dog walkers
✦ Having a dog reduces blood pressure and boosts the immune system
✦ Dog owners make fewer visits to their doctors
✦ And dog owners are likely to recover faster from heart attacks

The research confirms that owning a dog has benefits for both physical and psychological health.[22] Scientists in Japan report that dog owners get a surge of the 'love drug', the bonding hormone oxytocin, when playing with their pets, which lowers stress and wards off depression.[23]

The ones to read
Social Intelligence: The New Science of Human Relationships by Daniel Goleman
Love 2.0 by Barbara Fredrickson

CHAPTER 10

Vitality: The Body–Mind Connection

✦ **What is it?** The link between physical and mental health.
✦ **Try this for:** Energy, positive emotions.
✦ **If you like this, try also:** Meditation (Chapter 6) and Positive Directions (Chapter 12).

Psychology can sometimes give the impression of being a science that ignores what's going on beneath the neck and yet the body is one of the most powerful resources you have available – for free – to overcome depression. Physical activity does much, if not more, of what an anti-depressant can do to replenish levels of serotonin (to help with motivation and willpower) and norepinephrine (to increase focus and attention). Plus you get the reward of a dopamine hit, activating the brain's pleasure circuits.[1] Exercise is a highly effective natural anti-depressant.

There is much greater awareness now of the holistic nature of well-being and how the body can influence the mind in positive ways, which is known as somatopsychic wellness. Mental well-being is built on the foundations of good physical health. Sleep, diet, exercise, relaxation – they all have an impact on whether you feel up or down. Serious or chronic health conditions can trigger a downward spiral. Depression saps your vitality, but the body can be used as an instrument to restore your energy and recover your well-being.

Get moving

When you're depressed it can seem like a super-human effort to summon up an optimistic thought or to experience the mildest of positive emotions. This is where physical activity is your friend. Moving your body produces endorphins, feel-good hormones, which lift the mood naturally, so that you're more able to think positively. That's why I regard physical activity as a way of kick-starting your upward spiral on the back of a release of endorphins. This helps you get into a better mental space, which makes it easier to engage with the other practices in this book.

The challenge is to find a form of physical activity that you can persuade yourself to do. Depression is demotivating as well as de-energizing, so you need to make it small and manageable. That might mean a short walk down the road, dancing around your kitchen table to your favourite music (even three minutes can have a positive effect), or five minutes outdoors working in the garden. Notice how your mood begins to shift as you start to move physically. It is also a distraction from brooding, and can even be a catalyst for creativity. If I get stuck trying to figure something out, I find I am able to solve it as I walk.

The key is to find a physical activity that feels like a pleasure rather than a punishment. For Prof Michael Argyle, author of *The Psychology of Happiness*, that was Scottish country dancing, which had the additional pluses of being sociable and to music. What works for you? Here are some easy ways to get started on being physical:

✦ Walking
✦ Swimming
✦ Cycling
✦ Jogging
✦ Yoga
✦ Martial arts
✦ Gardening
✦ Dancing

Another clue as to which physical activity to choose is to think of what puts you into 'flow', that state of total immersion where you're completely absorbed in what you're doing. Sportspeople call it being 'in the zone' but you can also find it in activities such as gardening or the martial arts. What do you lose yourself in?

Physical activity has such benefits for mental health that Harvard psychologist Dr Tal Ben-Shahar famously said that not exercising is like taking depressants.

Physical activity ...

✦ Boosts mood through the release of endorphins
✦ Alleviates stress and anxiety
✦ Increases self-confidence and a sense of control
✦ Distracts from negative thoughts and emotions
✦ Encourages social interaction

Exercise is frequently prescribed as a treatment for depression and it can also prevent relapse. One American study compared the effects of exercise, anti-depressants and a combination of both on people with major depression. All three groups showed significant improvements, but six months after the experiment ended, the people who had recovered in the group who used exercise had significantly lower relapse rates than those in the medication group. Continuing to exercise reduced the likelihood of a further diagnosis of depression. Exercise has been shown to be one of the best forms of depression treatment.[2]

Green exercise – physical activity outdoors in nature – is particularly good for mental health. Even just five minutes of exercise in a green space boosts well-being.[3] Spending time in 'blue spaces', such as by the sea, a river or lake, can also have a positive effect on mental health, particularly in terms of stress reduction. Here are some suggestions to make physical activity a part of your recovery:

✦ Make it **easy**. Go for small steps, rather than attempting something too ambitious, which might stop you doing it again.
✦ Make it **every day**. Incorporate physical activity into your daily life: walk instead of drive; take the stairs; turn the housework into a workout.
✦ Make it **sociable**. Find an exercise buddy – by having someone alongside you, you have twice the motivation to draw upon.
✦ Make it a **habit**. Exercise for someone who is prone to depression is rather like a daily shot of insulin for a diabetic – something you need to do every day but which is, ultimately, a lifesaver.

Rest and renewal

Remember when people had 'spare time'? When Sundays were a day of rest rather than a day to catch up? The boundaries between work and play have become blurred. You're never really off duty. Smartphones mean that you're always accessible, even when you're on holiday. Modern lifestyles barely acknowledge the need for rest and renewal. It's a way of life that disturbs the balance needed for well-being.

My first experience of major depression came after a period where I was regularly working 60-hour weeks as a radio producer. On the outside I was successful, but on the inside I was very stressed, on the go all the time and surviving on a diet of caffeine and sugary snacks. If I wasn't at work, I was thinking about work. I never switched off and eventually the inevitable happened – burnout. When you ignore the body's need for renewal, you risk becoming depleted. Life becomes empty and flat. Classic signs of burnout are low mood, feeling disillusioned and lack of energy. The door opens to depression.

Pause for renewal

Rest may be an unfashionable word in our fast-paced world, but without it there is no renewal and your mental health is at risk. Maintaining a balance between activity and renewal is important as too much of either leads to sub-optimal living. It helps to tune into the body's messages, which let us know when things are getting out of balance. If you have too much of one thing and not enough of something else, you'll hear a voice of complaint inside. Listening is about paying attention to your needs, whether it's for rest, renewal or more variety in life. It's easy to disregard these messages – this came home to me in the process of writing this chapter alongside my day job. I was ignoring signs that life was getting out of balance until I was stopped in my tracks by an injury, which triggered an illness. That's when I finally got the message, except by then, of course, it was too late – my physical downturn in health was followed by a psychological one. I wish now that I'd paid attention to those messages telling me to rest and renew.

Applying the brake

The autonomic nervous system, which regulates our internal organs, has two main branches. The sympathetic nervous system (SNS) is the body's accelerator, the stress response, which primes us for 'fight or flight' when we face a threat. This is the adrenaline mode that pumps you up so that you can take action. The trouble is that many of us live our lives stuck in the SNS. The modern workplace depends on it. The parasympathetic nervous system (PNS), on the other hand, is the brake that triggers the 'rest-and-digest' response and other processes that happen when the body is in a state of relaxation. This is the route to renewal. How is your balance between the two?

If you tend to crash and burn, then your body is probably shouting at you to take it easy for a change. Renewal involves self-care: attending to your needs; restocking your reserves whether by resting, sleeping, good nutrition, physical exercise, getting out into nature, taking a break, doing something different or having a change of scene. All of these actions will make deposits into your energy bank.

Energy: the fuel of happiness

Energy is a precious resource in the 21st century, not only as the fuel that powers our world, but also the personal energy that makes it possible to engage with life. And engagement is, according to Martin Seligman, one of three pathways to authentic happiness alongside pleasure and meaning. Energy and emotions are connected. A peak emotion such as joy is often matched by a burst of energy. Conversely, when your energy is down, your mood tends to follow suit. Feeling depressed, hopeless or defeated are states that are low in both emotion and energy. One of the characteristics of depression is the way it strips away every ounce of energy, leaving in its place a lethargy, from which it is hard to muster any kind of motivation to do anything.

Whereas depression depletes us of positive emotions, energy provides the fuel for happiness. It is useful, therefore, to understand more about the nature of energy. One principle of energy is that it diminishes both with overuse and underuse. You need a balance between expending energy and renewing it. Unfortunately, the need for recovery is often viewed as a sign of weakness. In *The Power of Full Engagement*,[4] the authors Loehr and Schwartz suggest that we think of energy as a series of sprints rather than a marathon. A sprinter will engage powerfully for a short period, have their eye on the finishing line and then they'll rest before their next exertion. But a marathon runner keeps going on and on until they drop. The recommendation is to live your life as a series of sprints – fully engaging for a period of time and then disengaging for renewal before jumping back into the arena. Another principle of energy is that you need to stretch it beyond your normal limits to build it up. This is how you grow the 'muscle' for energy, developing strength and flexibility as you go.

I noticed this when I turned to swimming to help my recovery from depression. The first steps were simply to get myself to the pool with the greatest of ease. That meant taking the easy route of driving myself there and committing to no more than getting into the pool. Aim to do something small rather than setting the bar so high that it puts you off trying again. Having discovered that it was actually quite enjoyable to go for a swim, each time I pushed myself to do an extra lap. Very soon I was able to increase the distance I could swim and my vitality grew. The key is to make it really easy so that you actually do it, take the time to recover and then stretch yourself a bit further. You can develop 'muscle' in other areas, too, such as optimism. For example, the more you practise exercises such as the 'best possible self' (*see* p130), the stronger and more authentic you will eventually become in your capacity for optimism.

Besides physical energy, there are also emotional, mental and spiritual energies, which can be developed in the same way that you build physical energy. So, stretch each type beyond its usual limits – by then its functional capacity will be reduced, but after a period of recovery, it will be stronger than before and more capable of handling the next challenge. All these forms of energy share the same characteristics when they're functioning well: strength, endurance, flexibility and resilience. They are all connected, leading into downward or upward spirals. So an energy-draining scenario might be one where you feel pessimistic about the future of the job you're in (emotional energy-drainer) and you waste a lot of time worrying about it (mental energy-drainer), so you comfort-eat mindlessly (physical energy-drainer), and so on downward.

An example of an upward spiral could be when you start walking to work and feel better for it (physical energy-booster) and your increased physical well-being then leads to you feeling more optimistic about life (emotional energy-booster). With this increased energy you begin to think more creatively about how to improve your work situation (mental energy-booster) and as you put them into action, you discover a new direction, which gives you greater meaning in life (spiritual energy-booster). You're into a virtuous cycle where one form of energy stimulates another.

Food for mood

It's a simple equation – what you eat affects how you feel. Good nutrition supports your emotional well-being. Your diet can have a positive influence on your brain chemistry, and the way you eat, such as making sure you have regular meals, can maintain your mood. Improving your diet will help you think more clearly and to have more positive feelings and calmer moods. You will feel better and have more vitality. The message is a familiar one – a nutritious, balanced diet contains lots of fresh fruit and vegetables (at least five portions a day), as well as lean proteins and complex carbohydrates. Think about vitamin and mineral supplements, because the soil that produces our food is increasingly depleted of essential nutrients. Consult a dietician or nutritionist for advice tailored to your needs.

Eating for happiness: feed the brain

✦ **Vitamin B** Low levels of B-complex vitamins are common culprits for mild depression. Unfortunately, they can't be stored in the body so you need them in your daily diet or a B-complex supplement. **Folic acid** (aka **Vitamin B$_9$**) is found in leafy vegetables such as spinach and broccoli and is used to fortify cereals and bread. Good sources of **Vitamin B$_6$** include meat, fish, wholegrain produce, vegetables, nuts and bananas. **Vitamin B$_{12}$** is found in eggs, dairy produce, meat, poultry and fish.

✦ **Vitamin C** Keep up your intake of Vitamin C, which is known to be a mood elevator.

✦ **Vitamin D** Low levels of the sunshine vitamin are linked to depression symptoms and fatigue. Egg yolks, salmon and tuna are a food source. Sunlight absorbed through the skin helps your brain to make serotonin, the neurotransmitter that plays a significant role in elevating the mood and managing SAD (Seasonal Affective Disorder).

✦ **Serotonin** To make this feel-good neurotransmitter, the body needs **tryptophan**, an amino acid. This is present in most protein-based food. You find it in poultry, red meat, fish, eggs, beans, peanuts, seeds, oats, yogurt, cottage cheese, chickpeas, bananas and chocolate (don't get too excited – chocolate's benefits lie in a *moderate* consumption of the 70 percent dark chocolate variety). **5-HTP** (5-hydroxytryptophan) is another amino acid involved in the production of serotonin, which is available as a dietary supplement.

✦ **Minerals** Low mineral levels are linked to low mood. **Magnesium** is nature's chill pill and an antidote to stress, calming down the nervous system. Whole grains, beans, leafy green veggies and nuts are good sources, or take a bath in Epsom salts (magnesium sulphate). A deficiency of **selenium** is linked to depression and raising levels of it improves mood; find it in Brazil nuts, meat, fish, eggs and spinach. **Zinc** helps the body deal with stress and low levels are a marker for depression. Major food sources of zinc are meat, poultry, dairy, oysters, beans and nuts.

✦ **Complex carbohydrates** These have a calming effect. Carbohydrates provide the energy that fuels the body and they also help to produce serotonin. Your brain experiences a mild tranquilizing effect when you eat carbs – think of how comforting a plate of pasta or potatoes is when stress levels are high. Carbs calm the nerves, which is why many people turn to them when depressed or anxious. They are nature's chill pill. Choose **complex carbs** such as wholegrain pasta, bread, brown rice, legumes and beans that release their energy slowly for a longer-lasting effect.

✦ **Water** The brain is about 85 percent water. Optimal brain functioning depends on having enough hydration to keep the brain signals moving. Water supplies energy to the brain; its cells require more energy than most other cells in the body. Water also facilitates the movement of the feel-good neurotransmitters serotonin and dopamine as well as removing feel-bad toxins from the body. The brain has no way of storing water, which means there's a risk of dehydration if you don't drink water regularly, so drink, drink, drink! Dehydration is associated with fatigue and negative moods – some experts believe there to be a link between dehydration and depression.

What to avoid

✦ **Simple sugars** These stress the body. Refined carbohydrates are those found in many processed products, in sweet foods and those made of white flour, such as bread, cakes, pastries and biscuits. What happens is that you get a spike in blood sugar levels; eating **refined carbs** produces a sugar high, but then this is followed by crashing into a low, as insulin rushes to deal with the excess of sugar. This can leave you feeling even worse than before, with a drop in mood and energy. Fast-releasing sugars also stimulate the release of cortisol, a stress hormone, into the bloodstream.

✦ **Caffeinated drinks** Caffeine works by stimulating the central nervous system – often too much, especially if you are sensitive to it – which aggravates anxiety disorders, interferes with sleep, increases levels of the stress hormone cortisol and causes rapid fluctuations in blood-sugar levels. These are all factors that can worsen the symptoms of depression. Many people regard caffeine as a pick-me-up, but for people who are prone to depression, it can make the symptoms worse so it is advisable to cut back on it.

Breathe

In moments of anxiety my go-to tool is a simple one – deep breathing. As you breathe out it puts the brakes on the body and activates the parasympathetic nervous system. Intentional breathing practices can:

✦ Reduce depression and anxiety
✦ Strengthen the ability to regulate emotions
✦ Increase happiness and optimism
✦ Improve trauma symptoms
✦ Reduce impulsivity, cravings and addictions
✦ Improve sleep

Laugh

Something happens to people as they grow older. They become more serious as they take on responsibilities and the joy of childhood is lost. Laughter is a powerful way to bring that lightness back. It has the ability to shift your mood in an instant and has benefits for physical health too – lowering blood pressure, increasing tolerance of pain and boosting the immune system. Laughter is a good stressbuster – simply anticipating having a laugh can stimulate the production of mood-boosting endorphins. Enjoy the therapeutic benefits of laughter by watching comedies, hanging out with friends with a good sense of humour, or try 'laughter yoga', a practice originating in India where people come together to laugh their way to better well-being.

The ones to read
The Power of Full Engagement by Jim Loehr and Tony Schwartz
Positive Psychology and the Body by Kate Hefferon

CHAPTER 11

From Strength to Strength: You at Your Best

♦ **What is it?** The positive self and your inner resources.

♦ **Try this for:** Energy, positive emotions, well-being and success.

♦ **If you like this, try also:** Positive Directions (Chapter 12).

Depression acts as the very opposite of strengths. Strengths represent the presence of well-being. They provide a source of energy that helps you function well and puts you on the path to flourishing, whereas depression is enfeebling, leaving you all too aware of your weaknesses. No surprise then that it is easy to lose sight of your strengths and of how these assets can support you on the journey out of depression. They point you toward a direction in life that is right for you (more on which in the next chapter). Your strengths strengthen you. They provide you with the energy to recover your well-being. People who actively use their strengths are more confident, happy, productive, resilient and satisfied with life. They enjoy greater well-being and success. Your strengths are the key to realizing your potential. The cherry on the cake is that when you use your strengths, you're on your way to excelling with ease because it's something that comes naturally to you!

Positive psychology is often referred to as the science of strengths, because they make up the positive side of who we are. The study of strengths has rebalanced the field of psychology, which was accused of being overly focused on what is wrong with people rather than what is right. Prof Alex Linley, co-author of *The Strengths Book*, defines a strength as a particular way of behaving, thinking or feeling which enables optimal performance that is both authentic and energizing.[1] If it makes you feel good, you perform well, are energized, in flow and have a sense of 'yes this is the real me', then it is a strength. There are two types of strength:

✦ **Personal strengths** also called character or signature strengths – positive qualities like perseverance, courage or kindness.
✦ **Performance strengths** – your talents, such as problem-solving or the gift of persuasion.

Strengths are relevant in both personal and professional development. They help you function well at work and in life. Strengths are also major ingredients in resilience – they strengthen you to keep going during times of adversity. Your strengths hold a treasure trove of benefits for your well-being[2] because they:

+ Generate optimism
+ Develop confidence
+ Encourage insight
+ Produce positive emotions
+ Help to achieve goals
+ Build resilience
+ Protect against mental illness
+ Provide a sense of direction

The strengths approach is at the core of positive psychology coaching and positive psychotherapy. In coaching, strengths act as levers that you can pull to help you perform well and achieve your goals. In psychotherapy, taking a strengths approach enables the therapist to gain a wider and more integrated understanding of their client – their strengths as well as their symptoms. These are the inner resources that you can draw on to overcome depression, or as Dr Tayyab Rashid, co-creator of positive psychotherapy puts it, 'strengths can be marshalled to undo troubles'. One of the early studies in positive psychology tested a range of practices and discovered that finding new ways of using strengths leads to higher happiness and lower levels of depression symptoms six months down the line.[3] Using your strengths sets up a virtuous cycle – you perform well, which in turn generates positive emotions, overcomes the negativity bias and puts you on track for success. The benefits of using your strengths accumulate and can help you to move from a state of languishing into flourishing. One of the core principles of positive psychology is that your greatest potential for growth lies in developing your strengths rather than fixing your weaknesses. So this is where to focus your efforts to get the maximum return.

We are often reluctant to talk about our strengths, preferring to focus on shortcomings instead. Many of us find it hard to even recognize them. If we're naturally good at something, we often assume everyone else must find it easy, too. Not true! We tend to undervalue our strengths rather than take a pride in them. Your self-esteem will grow as you invest in your strengths – it helps to build confidence and overcomes a negative self-image.

The virtuous cycle of strengths

Using your strengths often

Increases positive emotions and develops confidence

Overcomes the negativity bias

Improves performance and leads to flourishing

Activating your strengths

✦ Begin drawing up a list of your strengths. You might include positive qualities such as kindness, compassion, fairness, a caring nature, common sense, leadership, etc.

✦ Add the things you're naturally good at, that energize you or put you into flow, such as design, communication, music, cooking, nurturing, etc.

✦ Ask friends and relatives what they think your strengths are.

✦ Return to the list whenever you think of something to add.

✦ You might want to keep the list in your journal or some other place where you can savour your strengths.

✦ When you have your list make a plan to use your strengths more. Choose a particular strength each day or week, and put it into action.

✦ Once you've made a habit of using your strengths, look for new opportunities to apply them in. This is the route to a sustainable increase in well-being.

How to identify your strengths

Now that you are aware of the merits of getting to know your strengths, it's good to get into a habit of spotting strengths in yourself and others. On the following page is a checklist to help you identify when your strengths might be in play.

STRENGTHS-SPOTTING CHECKLIST[4]

Your Best: What are you doing when you are at your best?

Ease: What do you find easy and what are you naturally good at?

Energy: When do you feel at your most alive? What energizes you?

Authenticity: What makes you say 'this is the real me'?

Fast Learner: What sort of skill do you pick up rapidly and effortlessly?

Motivation: What do you do just for the love of it?

Focus: What are you naturally drawn to? What attracts your attention?

Flow: What puts you 'in the zone' where you're completely absorbed and lose track of time?

Passion: What are you passionate about? What do you get animated talking about?

Childhood: What were you good at as a child? How does it show up in your life now?

The guide to human strengths

Bravery, integrity, compassion, persistence, humility, forgiveness, fairness, gratitude, open-mindedness …

Wouldn't it be good to have a comprehensive guide to all of humanity's positive characteristics? One of the major achievements in positive psychology has been to do just that. *The Character Strengths and Virtues*[5] handbook and classification is the result of a landmark research project to survey and document what is best about people. It's a manual of mental wellness, in effect, the opposite of the DSM (the *Diagnostic and Statistical Manual of Mental Disorders*), the classification that psychiatrists refer to in diagnosing mental illness. The 24 distinct character strengths are universally valued. Each strength belongs in one of six groups or 'virtues' – wisdom, courage, humanity, justice, temperance and transcendence. By investing in developing the strength you gain the virtue. So, for example, if you have character strengths of creativity, curiosity, love of learning, open-mindedness or perspective and you invest in developing them, you will gain the virtue of wisdom. If you have a strength in kindness or love, then you can develop the virtue of humanity. The chart on the following four pages lists all 24 character strengths, which everyone has in various degrees. You can take the test for free and find out the order of your 24 at www.viasurvey.org.

THE VALUES IN ACTION (VIA) CLASSIFICATION OF CHARACTER STRENGTHS

WISDOM – cognitive strengths that are about acquiring and applying knowledge.

- **Creativity** (originality, ingenuity): You enjoy thinking of new ways to do things, including artistic achievement and innovation.

- **Curiosity** (interest, novelty-seeking, openness to experience): You like exploration and discovery, finding new subjects and topics fascinating.

- **Judgment and Open-mindedness** (critical thinking): You think things through and examine them from all sides, not jumping to conclusions, weighing all evidence fairly, being able to change your mind in light of the evidence.

- **Love of Learning**: You have a passion for mastering new skills, topics and bodies of knowledge.

- **Perspective** (wisdom): People who know you consider you wise. You are able to provide wise counsel to others and have ways of looking at the world that make sense to yourself/others.

COURAGE – emotional strengths that involve the exercise of will to accomplish goals in the face of opposition, external or internal.

- **Bravery** (valour): You do not shrink from threat, challenge, difficulty or pain, speaking up for

→

what's right even if there's opposition, acting on convictions even if unpopular.

- **Perseverance** (persistence, industriousness): You work hard to finish what you start, persevering in a course of action in spite of obstacles, 'getting it out the door', taking pleasure in completing tasks.

- **Honesty** (authenticity, integrity): You live your life in a genuine and authentic way, speaking the truth and acting sincerely, taking responsibility for your feelings and actions.

- **Zest** (vitality, enthusiasm, vigour, energy): You approach everything you do with excitement and energy, not doing things half-heartedly, living life as an adventure, feeling alive and activated.

HUMANITY – interpersonal strengths that involve tending to and befriending others.

- **Love** (capacity to love and be loved): You value close relations with others, in particular those where sharing and caring are reciprocated; being close to people.

- **Kindness** (generosity, nurturance, care, compassion, altruistic love): You are kind, generous and nice to others.

- **Social Intelligence** (emotional intelligence, personal intelligence): You know how to fit into different social situations, being aware of the motives/feelings of yourself and others, knowing what makes other people tick.

JUSTICE – civic strengths that underlie healthy community life.

- **Teamwork** (citizenship, social responsibility, loyalty): You excel as a member of a group, being loyal to the team, doing your share.

- **Fairness**: You treat all people fairly, not letting feelings bias decisions about others, giving everyone a fair chance.

- **Leadership**: You excel at encouraging a group to get things done and maintain good relations within the group, leading group activities.

TEMPERANCE – strengths that protect against excess.

- **Forgiveness and Mercy**: You forgive those who have done you wrong, accepting others' shortcomings, giving people a second chance, not being vengeful.

- **Humility**: You do not seek the spotlight and others reognize and value your modesty.

- **Prudence**: You are a careful person not taking undue risks, not saying or doing things that might later be regretted.

- **Self-Regulation** (self-control): You are a disciplined person, controlling your appetites and emotions.

TRANSCENDENCE – strengths that forge connections to the universe and provide meaning.

→

- **Appreciation of Beauty and Excellence** (awe, wonder, elevation): You notice and appreciate beauty and excellence in all domains of life, from nature to art to science to everyday experience.

- **Gratitude**: You are aware of and thankful for the good things that happen, taking time to express thanks.

- **Hope** (optimism, future-mindedness, future orientation): You expect the best in the future and work to achieve it.

- **Humour** (playfulness): You like to laugh and tease, bringing smiles to other people is important to you; seeing the light side, making (not necessarily telling) jokes.

- **Spirituality** (faith, purpose): Your beliefs shape your actions and are a source of comfort to you. You have coherent beliefs about the higher purpose and meaning of the universe, knowing where you fit within the larger scheme.

Used by permission of the VIA Institute on Character (c) 2017

You may be interested to know that people who've recovered from a psychological disorder tend to have appreciation of beauty, creativity, curiosity, gratitude and love of learning among their top strengths. Those who recover from a serious physical illness have higher appreciation of beauty, bravery, curiosity, fairness, forgiveness, gratitude, humour, kindness, love of learning and spirituality.[6]

Completing the strengths test is one of the most rewarding things you can do for your well-being.

✦ What are your top five strengths?
✦ Which 'virtues' do your top five belong to?
✦ Do your top strengths cluster in any particular virtue?
✦ What new ways can you think of to use your top strengths?

There are no right or wrong answers here, this is about getting to know your strengths and appreciating them as assets. I've witnessed transformations as a result of taking a strengths test. On one memorable occasion I was coaching a teenager who was a heavy user of drugs. Danni* had little aspiration; she thought she'd probably end up in prison just like her older brothers. That's what everyone told her. She took the test and discovered that her strengths are concentrated in the virtue of humanity – love, kindness and emotional intelligence. This was no surprise to her, as she was the peacemaker in her family and could relate well to young children. But having official confirmation of her strengths lit a fire within her. She started attending college regularly, she cut back and then gave up the drugs and got herself some work experience. She turned a corner in her life. Having had a pessimistic view of her future, she saw that she didn't have to end up on the same path as her brothers. She now had a goal – to

*Name changed

become a youth worker – which played to her strengths and was aligned with who she really was. As she began to apply her strengths, her confidence soared and life changed. She went through a metamorphosis from teen druggie into a dynamic young woman.

That is an experience of someone at the start of their working life. I've also seen the benefits of taking a strengths-based approach to changing career in mid-life. Knowing your strengths can clarify your choice of direction and help you to make the change from a position of strength with the energy, confidence and motivation to make it happen.

Applying the strong to what's wrong

Your strengths support your psychological well-being and protect against mental illness. Optimism, for example, prevents depression and anxiety. Other strengths such as courage, future-mindedness, relationship-building, faith, a work ethic, hope, honesty and perseverance are also known to protect against mental illness.[7] Using your strengths generates positive emotions, and this, in turn, builds resilience so that you're more able to cope with life's trials and bounce back from them.

In therapy getting to know your strengths serves a double purpose, firstly by helping you see yourself in a more positive light (something that gets lost in depression), and secondly as tools you can use on your journey to recovery. Dr Tayyab Rashid, co-creator of positive psychotherapy[8], asks clients to write a Positive Introduction – a real-life story that shows them at their best or during a peak moment in their lives, illustrating some of their top strengths in action. I've used this technique in groupwork and found it to be a powerful way of helping people appreciate their strengths and have those strengths reflected back to them.

When you're at a low ebb, your strengths can help make things a little easier. Finding ways of using them gives you evidence of things that you *are* good at and boosts your confidence. Your strengths can be applied to build positives and reduce the negatives in life. Here are some coaching activities that will help you to make the most of your strengths. This is something that you could do in a coaching session or working with a friend.

A TOOLKIT OF STRENGTHS

Strengths Story: Tell the story of each of your top strengths. When did you first notice that you had this strength? How does it show up in your life now? What are the advantages of having the strength?
Discuss situations where it's been helpful to have this strength. Include examples from your life that illustrate your strengths in action.

New Ways to Use Strengths: Think of new ideas to apply each of your top five character strengths. Then, commit to some dates on which to try using one or more of your strengths in a new way.

→

Strengths Solution: Take a real-life issue that you're facing at the moment and see how you might be able to apply each of your top five strengths to find a new way of tackling the problem. Ask yourself, '*How might my strength in .... help solve the problem of ....?*' What new ideas or insights do you gain to address the problem? This is a good one to do with someone else who may spot things you miss.

Goals: Choose one of your life goals. Now apply each of your top five VIA strengths in turn to see how it may help to reach the goal. Again, ask yourself, '*How might my strength in .... help achieve the goal of ....?*'

Strengths at work

Your strengths also hold your potential for success in the workplace. The research shows that people who are able to craft their work around their strengths are more engaged in what they do, perform better and enjoy greater success in their roles. People who have the opportunity to focus on their strengths every day are six times more likely to be engaged with their jobs and more than three times as likely to report having an excellent quality of life.[9] It bears repeating that using your strengths in your work is the way to **excel with ease**, because you'll be performing well at something that comes naturally to you. So invest in developing your strengths rather than in fixing your weaknesses. This represents a paradigm shift for the workplace, where training is traditionally geared toward developing areas of weakness rather than strength. When you focus on weaknesses there's a ceiling to what you can achieve, because it's something you're not naturally good at. The best you can achieve is mediocrity. But when you focus on developing your strengths, there are no such limits. This is how you are when you're at your strongest and fulfilling your potential. Incidentally, the advice for your areas of weakness is to put in enough effort to master the necessities involved but to channel your efforts instead into your strengths. That is where you will get the best return.

If you're at a crossroads in life, your top strengths will provide you with a strong clue as to which way to move forward. I've seen people turn a corner in their lives when they begin to follow their strengths. It's particularly helpful if you are thinking of a new career. One of my key strengths is curiosity, which I drew on extensively in an earlier career in the media. Whenever I went to interview someone, my strength of curiosity had me brimming with questions. I carried this strength together with social intelligence, also in my top five, into my work as a psychologist and coach. Curiosity and social intelligence enable me to find out what makes people tick and get to the heart of the matter with speed and ease. Your strengths are like a bundle of talents you can take from one career into the next, applying them in new ways.

The shadow side is that it is possible to overplay your strengths. Using them to excess or misapplying them can lead to a loss of performance and things going wrong. That's when you begin to see the shadow side of a strength. Humour overdone can miss its mark or appear as a lack of respect. Leadership taken too far can alienate the people around you. Creativity overdone can lead to many projects started at the expense of those completed. The 'golden mean' is to use the right strength in the right amount in the right place and at the right time. Think of it as dialling it up or down as the situation requires.

The bottom 80

We live in a society that has traditionally rated academic achievement highly as the path to a happy and thriving life. This narrow definition of success is given to children at an early age, generating anxiety about whether they are good enough to make the grade. One of the beauties of the strengths approach is that it celebrates broader talents beyond academic ones and this is especially relevant for young people. I've worked with teenagers who've dropped out of education and had zero belief in being good at anything besides a talent for getting into trouble. Helping disaffected young people to identify their strengths builds self-confidence based on something concrete rather than empty affirmations and gives them a means to reconnect with society. Christine Duvivier, a positive psychologist from Boston, has studied the talents of the 'bottom 80 percent', that is those of the majority rather than the elite.[10] She challenges many of the myths associated with education, for example the myth that being a top student leads to a great life and if you're not means you're not intelligent, hardworking or gifted.

Many capabilities are not nurtured within the existing model of education; talents such as the entrepreneurial spirit, manual dexterity, the visual eye or the art of persuasion, which is so critical to sales and marketing. The message to take away from this is that many of our strengths may not be recognized early in life and may not fit the mould of what's conventionally considered to be a strength, but they hold the seeds of success that can be developed at any stage, whether at the start of working life, in mid-life or in retirement. Your strengths point you toward a fresh new direction, which is the subject of the next chapter.

The ones to read

Average to A+: Realising Strengths in Yourself and Others by Alex Linley

Character Strengths and Virtues: A Handbook and Classification by Christopher Peterson and Martin Seligman

CHAPTER 12

Positive Directions: Moving Forward

✦ **What is it?** 'Eudaimonic' well-being – a deeper happiness, functioning well and realizing your potential.

✦ **Try this for:** The future, life purpose, setting goals and a new chapter after depression.

✦ **If you like this, try also:** Strengths (Chapter 11).

In this final chapter I'd like to invite you to make plans for a life beyond the lows. One of the common features of depression is looking back and ruminating over how things went wrong, how you suffered a setback or trauma, or how life didn't turn out quite the way that you planned. You cannot change the past, but you can influence the shape of your future. Maybe the time has come for you to draw a line under that chapter of your life and begin anew.

Depression can be a signal that your current lifestyle is no longer working well for you and a sign that something has to change. In my own case it wasn't until I'd experienced several episodes of depression that I finally realized that I was on the wrong career path. Having made the changes I am much happier; I play to my strengths and no longer suffer from the crippling lows that once had me in their grip. The good news is that the past is not necessarily an indicator of the future. You have a high degree of influence over how things turn out even if you have a belief that your life is subject to factors beyond your control, such as luck, fate, circumstances or other people). Perhaps it is time now to let go of past difficulty, to look forward to a future where you operate from a position of strength. There are tools in this chapter to help you move forward positively, in a direction that is right for you now and with a sense of purpose that is authentic to you, aligned to who you really are.

Positive psychology is a science with many different facets but it can be summarized as being about two fundamental things: **how to feel good** and **how to function well**. **Feeling good** is the more familiar part that we've focused on in earlier chapters – it's about experiencing a cheerful mood, an abundance of positive emotions and peak happiness. **Functioning well** relates to a deeper sense of well-being. It's how we are when we're playing to our strengths and realizing our potential. It's about having meaning and purpose, experiencing personal growth and fulfilment. This is 'eudaimonic' well-being (*see* p33), meaning living well and doing well, which is based on actualizing your true nature or 'daimon'. The original concept of this dates back to the Ancient Greek philosophers. It's a 'quieter' form of happiness, which many psychologists think leads to a greater satisfaction with life and a more sustainable well-being. In this chapter we look at some of the elements that make up this form of well-being and how we can have more of it.

The meaning of life

What gives your life meaning? Maybe your loved ones, your faith, a vocation, your achievements? Making a difference in the world? Perhaps it is creative expression or your journey of self-discovery? Whatever the source, it's a deeply personal matter. Big life events shape meaning, whether that's something positive, such as the birth of a child, or negative, in the case of surviving trauma. Life has meaning when there is a significance that goes beyond the momentary or the trivial, or when it has a purpose or coherence that transcends chaos.[1] Whichever the case, those who have a sense of meaning in life have better well-being than those who don't. A lack of meaning is one of the symptoms of depression. My last episode of depression came when I found that the meaning had gone from my life. Motherhood was the path I wanted to be on, but when it became clear that this was not going to happen (at least in the conventional sense) the black dog arrived. What really helped with recovery was to find a new purpose in life that was meaningful and motivating. My life purpose now is to help people onto the path to happiness and it is every bit as inspiring as when I first articulated it. It brings me great satisfaction when I fulfil my purpose in working with people. It delivers all the meaning in life that I need – and more.

We tend to find meaning in positive experiences, which provide us with a sense that things are as they are meant to be. Even simple pleasures can give meaning to life, such as a lazy sunny afternoon spent in the company of a loved one. On the other hand, we construct meaning from life's more difficult experiences as we try to make sense of what has happened. Viktor Frankl, the Austrian psychiatrist, wrote *Man's Search for Meaning*[2] about the time he spent incarcerated in a Nazi concentration camp. In the midst of his suffering and deprivation, Frankl describes an incident in which he was working in harsh, icy conditions and suddenly had a vision of his wife accompanied by a feeling of bliss. For him the revelation was that love gives life its greatest meaning. Even with nothing left in the world, it was still possible to experience meaning. Frankl suggests that meaning is found through these routes:

✦ Creating a work or carrying out a deed.
✦ Experiencing something or encountering someone.
✦ By the attitude we take toward unavoidable suffering.

One of the most potent ways of bringing meaning into your existence is to have a purpose in life, a sense of knowing what you're about and what you were born to do. Not only does it provide you with two of the three main pathways to authentic happiness – meaning and engagement[3] – but it also gives you a positive direction, a target for your energy and goals to aim for. Having a purpose gives your life a framework, which enables you to be more resilient to stresses and strain. Do you have a sense of your purpose? If not, you're not the only one. Many people feel little sense of purpose, wondering what they're meant to be doing with their lives and hesitating between many options, not knowing which to choose. Others doubt that there is a purpose in life for them. The big question is how do you find your purpose in life? Research suggests it comes about in one of three ways:[4]

✦ Being proactive, investing effort over time to clarify your life purpose.
✦ Through a transformative life event such as an illness or parenthood.
✦ Observing others and basing your purpose on what you learn from them.

So your life purpose is something you work toward, it arrives fully-formed or it emerges vicariously through your observation of other people. It can feel quite daunting to set about identifying something as significant as your purpose in life. Remember to keep a 'growth mindset' (*see* p21) about this – it is about trial and error, your purpose is not set in stone, but is something that can evolve over time and change throughout your life. There is often a deep sense of knowing when you connect with the purpose that is right for you. It feels congruent. Your body relaxes into it. Below are some activities that can help you to identify your life purpose, starting with one based on some of your most memorable life experiences.[5]

DISCOVERING YOUR LIFE PURPOSE – 1

Think of **three of the most positive, peak experiences** of your life:

1. ....

....

2. ....

....

3. ....

....

For the first one, ask yourself, '**What was important to me about this experience?**' Outline two reasons for each experience, writing a couple of sentences on each. Repeat for the other positive experiences. →

- ....

    ....

- ....

    ....

- ....

    ....

- ....

    ....

- ....

    ....

- ....

    ....

- When you've finished, underline the key words in each sentence. These relate to your core values.
- From this list select and **circle the three most important ones** to you.

→

- With this top three in mind, have a go at writing a simple **life purpose** statement. Play around with the order of the words until an idea of your life purpose emerges. Trust your gut instinct and keep going until you formulate a sentence that feels right for you. Have a guess if you're not sure.

My purpose in life is to...

....

....

....

Relax and enjoy the process. There is no right or wrong answer here. Your life purpose can change over time.

This exercise works well because it reveals your purpose in life via an indirect route. I've found it to be a powerful process to use with coaching clients, who often experience light-bulb moments as they formulate their life purpose. Once you've generated a purpose, notice if it is a good fit for you. Does it feel authentic and motivating? Having a new (or renewed) purpose will help you to move forward and is especially useful if you're at a career crossroads. Think of one small, manageable step that you could take toward living your life purpose. You might do some online research or make a phone call. Whatever it is, put a date in the diary and commit to taking that small step.

Next is another activity that can help you to get closer to identifying your source of meaning and purpose. Get yourself into a positive state beforehand to help the process – go for a walk, meditate, listen to music or spend some time in nature. This exercise involves writing, so you might want to use a journal to record your thoughts.

Positive legacy

✦ Think ahead to your life as you would like it to be and how you would prefer to be remembered by the people closest to you.
✦ What would you like them to say about you? What accomplishments and strengths would they mention?
✦ Allow yourself to daydream freely and give rein to your imagination. Try to keep it grounded in reality. Don't be too modest though – think big.
✦ Write a couple of paragraphs on your positive legacy.
✦ Put it away for a while. When you come to look at it again, notice what the themes are. What does it tell you about what gives meaning to your life? What clues does it give you about your purpose?
✦ Look back at what you've written and ask yourself the following questions: What can I do that is within my control to bring about my legacy? What am I currently doing that will move me closer to this goal?

Based on Chris Peterson's *A Primer in Positive Psychology*[6]

Depression is often linked to endings – a relationship, a job, a stage in life, a way of life. Painful as that is, once the mourning process is underway, endings can also pave the way for new beginnings. Having a goal is a major step in the recovery from depression, to help you move forward. My own experience of emerging from depression felt like the proverbial phoenix rising from the ashes. The old life had crashed and burned. It was time to find a new direction, although I tried my best to cling on to my old ways. One of the things that really helped was to focus on my strengths and how to use them to move into a new area. Your strengths point you toward a life purpose that is authentic and aligned with who you really are. Here is another activity to help you to identify your purpose, based on the strengths that you discovered in the previous chapter.

DISCOVERING YOUR LIFE PURPOSE – 2

Your strengths and other gifts are a clue to your vocation. Use this exercise to clarify a direction for applying your strengths.[7]

- Write a list of your top five character strengths from the VIA test.

  1. ....

  2. ....

  ➔

3. ....

4. ....

5. ....

- Write a list of around five other talents/gifts that you have – for example, you are artistic, sporty, musical, good with animals, make people laugh, have an eye for colour, etc.

    1. ....

    2. ....

    3. ....

    4. ....

    5. ....

- Write a list of things that make you angry in modern society (choose something that you might feel strongly enough to act upon).

    1. ....

    2. ....

    3. ....

    4. ....

    5. ....

→

Now pick one item from each category – whatever most attracts your attention from each list – and note them below.

a .... b ....

c ....

Use these three elements to formulate a life purpose statement as follows:

I'm going to take my strength in ....

and my gift for ....

to ....

(your anger expressed in the positive, as a call to action)*

Have a go – there is no right or wrong answer. If you don't know, guess!

* For example, if your anger is about the extent of mental illness in modern society, your statement expressed as a positive would be 'to promote psychological well-being' rather that 'to stop mental illness'.

Life rewards action

I hope you have more of an understanding now of eudaimonic well-being – the deeper well-being that arises from having meaning and purpose in life alongside a greater knowledge of your personal strengths and how you might draw on them to help you move forward. Depression is a debilitating condition and taking action can be the last thing you feel like doing. However, in order to move beyond being stuck you need to take action and that is when your life will begin to change. So here are some tips that can support you in turning a thought into a deed, which will help you to bring about a real change and live your life purpose.

A nudge in the right direction

✦ Taking many small steps is more likely to get the ball rolling rather than one big step. Set the bar low – foothills rather than mountains.

✦ Be kind to yourself and act in the moments when your mood is lighter. This could be after some physical or social activity.

✦ Take just one step a day. If there were a mantra to hold in mind it is this: try to do one small thing every day that takes you forward.

Goal-setting for change

The question at the heart of coaching is, 'What do you want?' This next section looks at what you would like for your life beyond the depression. What do you want to achieve? That might seem like an alien concept right now, but having a goal gives you a direction, something to aim for, and a purpose. There is ample research that shows that satisfaction with life comes through achieving goals that are important to you. Goal-setting is a mixed bag to someone in depression. Sometimes it is the failure to achieve your life goals that can act as a trigger to depression. This is especially the case in mid-life. Happiness tends to hit a low point in the mid-40s; realizing that it may be too late for you to achieve certain goals is a contributor to the mid-life crisis. But sometimes giving up on those long-held goals is what finally allows you to move forward. The good news is that after this mid-life dip happiness starts to rise again.[8]

I think it is best to hold goals lightly – view them more as intentions that give you a focus rather than as fixed points that you *must* achieve, where the failure to reach them might weigh heavily. My own happiness began to rise once I gave up on those long-held ambitions that I hadn't achieved and set intentions that were more flexible and that had a greater acceptance of what is. The following series of exercises are designed to help you obtain more clarity about the direction you want now for your life.

THE WHEEL OF WELL-BEING

This is a simple process to help you to work out which areas of your life need attention and where to focus your efforts to increase your well-being. Draw a circle or a wheel and divide it into eight segments. Label each part with an area of life – below is a list of some of the major areas of well-being, but feel free to include others that are significant for you.

- **Joy** – Fun, leisure and pleasure

- **Meaning** – Purpose, fulfilment, spirituality

- **Connection** – Relationships with loved ones, friends, others

- **Resilience** – Ability to deal with difficulty and bounce back

- **Vitality** – Physical health, energy, exercise

- **Personal Development** – Learning, self-expression

- **Work** – Career satisfaction

- ....

- ....

- ....

See an example of a Wheel of Well-being overleaf.

Your Wheel of Well-being

Label each section of the wheel with a life area. Then rate how satisfied you are with each area by drawing a line within the section. Score each area on a scale from 0 (very poor) to 10 (very good). The centre of the wheel is 0 and the outer edge is 10. A high score will place a line near the outer edge and a low score near the centre. You may want more space than is allocated here. If this is so, find a piece of blank paper and sketch out a larger wheel.

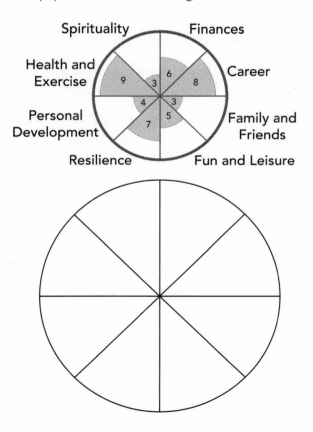

Once you've completed your Wheel of Well-being, ask yourself the following questions.

✦ How do you rate your well-being? What do you notice in your wheel?
✦ What is working well?
✦ What needs attention?
✦ Which area can you address now?
✦ What one small step could you take to make a big difference?

Copy each segment over into a Life-planning Chart like the one on p227. Then, set a goal for each area of life, making sure that you express it as an approach goal, that is, as something you want to move toward rather than an avoidant goal of something you want to escape from. Approach goals are more likely to be intrinsically motivating – something that you want to do for its own sake. Extrinsic motivation is when you are motivated to do something because it will bring you an external reward, such as money, better status, etc. Having an intrinsically motivating goal is more likely to inspire you to put the effort in and persist when the going gets tough.

Make sure that the thing you choose is a manageable goal. Think SMART – Specific, Measurable, Attainable, Relevant and with a Time-frame attached. The point of this is that if it is too big a target, the risk is that you might find it too daunting to tackle or give up once you run into obstacles and label yourself as a failure.

Keep the goal small enough to encourage yourself into action. Right now it's about moving off the starting block; you can take bigger steps a little further down the line when you feel ready for them. Your goal needs to be specific so that you have a real sense of what you're aiming for, such as going to the gym once a week rather than something general like 'to get fit'. Identify a first step toward the goal. Make sure it's easy, something that is well within your grasp. And then identify the next step.

With your goal in mind, consider your answer to the following questions, which will help you to further develop your vision:

✦ If I could wave a magic wand and give it to you right now, would you say yes without hesitation? If in doubt, then you may need to refine the goal further, so that the answer is a confident 'yes'.

✦ Get really specific about your goal. What is it you want? When? Where? Who else is involved?

✦ How might it come about? Be creative and generate as many options as you can think of.

✦ What resources would help you achieve your goal? People, organizations, books or websites?

✦ What will it be like when you achieve your goal? What evidence might you see? What might you hear? What will you feel? Use your senses to imagine how it will be – sights, sounds and feelings.

✦ Is the goal the right size to motivate you to take action? If it is too big, reduce it to something more

LIFE-PLANNING CHART

Life area ....

....

SMART goal ....

....

....

....

First step – make it easy ....

....

....

....

....

Next step ....

....

....

....

....

manageable. If it is too small, set the bar a bit higher so that you feel more inspired.

✦ Notice where you are on the journey to your goal. What progress has already been made?

✦ Adjust your goal, if necessary, to ensure that it is based on something within your control.

Here are a couple of questions that can help you prepare to take action and navigate around potential obstacles.

✦ What has to happen for you to achieve your goal?

✦ What's stopping you at the moment from reaching your goal?

Where there's a will, there's a way ...

Before we close I'd like to introduce you to hope, the more retiring cousin of optimism (*see* Chapter 7). Hope doesn't get the same attention as her more prominent relation, but nonetheless has something valuable to offer for the way ahead. Hope in positive psychology is much more than a belief in a positive outcome, it is a very practical concept. There are two parts to it: firstly, having the motivation to achieve goals (agency); and secondly, having a clear idea of how to get to the goals (pathways).[9] Hopelessness as a feeling is all too common in depression, but even if you don't *feel* hopeful about your goal, what the positive psychology version of hope offers is a concrete strategy to develop hopefulness and move toward your goal. This is the formula for hope:

1. Identify what you want (goals).

2. Think of a variety of routes toward your goal (pathways).

3. Apply yourself with energy to achieving that goal and keep going (agency).

With hope it's a case of where there's a will (agency), there's almost certainly a way (a pathway, in fact). What differentiates hopeful people from non-hopeful people is that when they find an obstacle on their route to a goal, they will be flexible and look for other pathways to get there. And this is where 'agency' comes into play, giving a hopeful person the energy and motivation to get started and to persist when the going gets tough. You may find it a struggle to be authentically hopeful, but here is a formula that removes the frustration and instead deconstructs hope into a series of steps that can take you on the way to your goal: from helplessness to hopefulness.

Happily ever after?
The maintenance diet

This book has explored evidence-based positive psychology practices which build happiness and help you recover your well-being. These tools can be used to boost your mood naturally, protect you from the downward spiral into depression and support you in overcoming a visit from the 'black dog'. Depression has many varied causes and your recovery will similarly benefit from taking a multi-faceted approach.

+ Practise gratitude and savouring to experience more positive emotions.
+ Practise optimism, the key tool in resilience.
+ Stay in touch with the people you value.
+ Focus on the physical foundations of well-being – energy, diet, exercise.
+ Reflect on the bigger picture – your meaning and purpose in life.
+ Use your strengths as levers to resolve problems and reach your goals.

Remember that while pleasure will give you the high of happiness in the moment, there is a deeper well-being that comes from having purpose in life and being engaged in activities that allow you to realize your potential. In a nutshell, eudaimonic well-being arises from the good feelings generated by engaging your strengths in the service of something meaningful.

'This too shall pass'

Optimists tend to react to the bad events in their lives by thinking that it is a temporary state of affairs. That 'this too shall pass'. Applying this optimism to depression, the positive news is that most episodes of depression have a life cycle and will run their course. The recovery from depression can feel slow – you may not even notice how the dark is receding while the light is increasing by degrees. Eventually there will be more frequent experiences of positive emotion and fewer days in the depths of despair.

The research indicates that once you've had an episode of depression, you're at a greater risk of having further episodes, hence the need for a maintenance diet of mood-boosting activities to keep the blues at bay. Look after your mental health and give it as much attention as you would your physical well-being. Simple everyday ways you can do that are by savouring the good things as they happen, practising the art of appreciation, reframing the negative and paying attention to the balance in your life between work, rest and play. Fill your reservoir of well-being with experiences that generate positive emotions or bring meaning into your life. This will build your resilience, help you to sail through the ups and downs and give you greater protection against depression when you next come to navigate the stormy waters of life.

Learn to recognize the signs that you might be heading into a downward spiral and use that as a cue to step up your practice of the techniques in the book. Apart from the occasional low mood, I now live life free from depression and my capacity for happiness is much greater than it has ever been. The same can happen for you, too. It is the practice that forms the neural connections that make a habit out of happiness. Things are more flexible than they are fixed. Life does change. Every cell in your body will renew itself. You can grow your happiness, increase your positivity, learn optimism even if you were a born pessimist and develop your strengths. There is a light at the end of the tunnel even if you don't believe it to be true. There is hope.

'Where there's life, there's hope.' *Cicero*

The one to read
Creating Your Best Life by Caroline Adams Miller, MAPP and Dr Michael Frisch

Chapter Notes

Preface

1 The Positive Psychology Center at the University of Pennsylvania (www.ppc.sas.upenn.edu)

2 Akhtar, M. (2017). *What is Post-Traumatic Growth?* London: Watkins Media Ltd

3 Hansen, K. (2018). Positive Psychology for Overcoming Symptoms of Depression: A Pilot Study Exploring the Efficacy of a Positive Psychology Self-Help Book versus a CBT Self-Help Book. *Behavioural and Cognitive Psychotherapy*

Chapter 1

1 Kaufmann, C., Boniwell, I. and Silberman, J. (2009). The Positive Psychology Approach to Coaching, in Bachkirova, T. and Cox, E. (eds) *The Sage Handbook of Coaching*, London: Sage Press

2 Seligman, M.E.P., Rashid, T., and Parks, A.C. (2006). Positive psychotherapy. *American Psychologist, 61*, 774–788

3 Berk, M. and Parker, G. (2009). The elephant on the couch: side-effects of psychotherapy, *Australian and New Zealand Journal of Psychiatry, 43*, 787–794

4 Lambert, M.J. (2004). Bergin and Garfield's *Handbook of Psychotherapy and Behaviour Change*. Chichester: Wiley, 5th edition

5 Akhtar M. and Boniwell, I. (2010). Applying positive psychology to alcohol-misusing adolescents: A group intervention. *Groupwork, 20* (3), 7–23

6 www.acss.org.uk/news/bulletins2013novembermtc9mentalwellbeing-htm/

7 Seligman, M.E.P., Rashid, T., and Parks, A.C. (2006). Positive psychotherapy. *American Psychologist, 61*, 774–788

8 Dweck, C.S. (2006). *Mindset: The New Psychology of Success.* New York: Random House

Chapter 2

1 Lyubomirsky, S., Sheldon, K.M., and Schkade, D. (2005). Pursuing happiness: The architecture of sustainable change. *Review of General Psychology, 9*, 111–131

2 Seligman, M.E.P. (2003) *Authentic Happiness* London, Nicholas Brealey Publishing; Lyubomirsky, S.(2007) *The How of Happiness.* London: Sphere

3 Seligman, op.cit.

4 Seligman, M.E.P. (2011). *Flourish.* London: Nicholas Brealey Publishing

5 Diener, E. (2000) Subjective Well-being: The science of happiness and a proposal for a national index. *American Psychologist, 55*, 56–67

6 Ryff, C.D. and Keyes, C.L.M. (1995) The structure of psychological well-being revisited. *Journal of Personality and Social Psychology, 69*, 719–27

7 Csikszentmihalyi, M. (1990). *Flow: The Psychology of Optimal Experience,* New York: Harper and Row

8 Ryan, R.M., and Deci, E.L. (2000). Self-determination

theory and the facilitation of intrinsic motivation, social development, and well-being. *American Psychologist, 55,* 68–78

9 Mauss, I.B., Tamir, M., Anderson, C.L., and Savino, N.S. (2011). Can seeking happiness make people happy? Paradoxical effects of valuing happiness. *Emotion,* 1–9

Chapter 3

1 Fredrickson, B.L. (2001). The role of positive emotions in positive psychology: The broaden-and-build theory of positive emotions. *American Psychologist, 56,* 218–26

2 Fredrickson, B.L. (2009). *Positivity.* New York: Crown Publishers

3 Frisch, M.B. (2006). *Quality of Life Therapy.* New Jersey: John Wiley and Sons

Chapter 4

1 Breathnach, S.B. (1996). *The simple abundance journal of gratitude.* New York: Warner

2 Lyubomirsky, S. (2007). *The How of Happiness.* London: Sphere Books

3 Lyubomirsky, S. (2007), op cit., p91

4 Emmons, R.A. & Shelton, C.M. (2005). Gratitude and the Science of Positive Psychology. In C.R. Snyder & S.J. Lopez (Eds.), *Handbook of Positive Psychology* (pp.459–471). London: Oxford University Press.

5 Seligman, M. E. P., Steen, T. A., Park, N., & Peterson, C. (2005). Positive psychology progress: Empirical validation of interventions. *American Psychologist,* 60, 410-421.

6 Pollay, D.J. (2008) Gratitude is a bridge to your positive future. Retrieved at positivepsychologynews.com/news/david-j-pollay/200811021119

7 Emmons, R. op.cit.

8 Gratitude: How to appreciate life's gifts (2010). Positive Psychology News Series.

9 Ibid.

10 For more on Appreciative Inquiry: Cooperrider, D.L., and Whitney, D. (2005). *Appreciative Inquiry: A positive revolution in change.* San Francisco: Berrett-Koehler Publishers

Chapter 5

1 Bryant, F.B. and Veroff, J. (2007). *Savoring: A new model of positive experiences.* Mahwah, N.J.: Lawrence Erlbaum Associates, Inc.

2 Honoré, C. (2005). *In Praise of Slow: How a Worldwide Movement is Challenging the Cult of Speed.* London, Orion Books

3 www.slowfood.com

4 Schooler, J.W., Ariely, D., and Loewenstein, G. (2003). The pursuit and assessment of happiness may be self-defeating. In I. Brocas and J.D. Carilloo (eds). *The psychology of economic decisions. Volume 1: Rationality and well-being* (pp.41–70) New York: Oxford University Press

5 Bryant and Veroff, op cit.

6 Diener, Sanvik and Pavot (1991). Happiness is the frequency, not the intensity of positive versus negative affect. In F. Strack, M. Argyle, and N. Schwarz (eds.), *Subjective well-being: An interdisciplinary*

perspective (pp.119–139). New York: Pergamon

7 Seligman, M.E.P, Rashid, T. and Parks, A.C. (2006) Positive psychotherapy. *American Psychologist* 61, pp.774–88

8 Boniwell, I., and Zimbardo, P. (2004). Balancing time perspective in pursuit of optimal functioning. In P.A. Linley and S. Joseph (eds.), *Positive psychology in practice.* New Jersey: John Wiley and Sons

9 Bryant, F.B., Smart, C.M., and King, S.P. (2005). Using the past to enhance the present: Boosting happiness through positive reminiscence. *Journal of Happiness Studies,* 6, 227–60

Chapter 6

1 Davidson, R.J., Kabat-Zinn, J., Schumacher, J., Rosenkranz, M., Muller, D., Santorelli, S.F., et al. (2003). Alterations in brain and immune function produced by mindfulness meditation. *Psychosomatic Medicine 65,* 564–70

2 Find out more about Davidson's work in the Lab for Affective Neuroscience at http://psyphz.psych.wise.edu

3 Hanh, T.N. (1991). *The Miracle of Mindfulness.* London, Rider Books

4 Davidson, R.J., Kabat-Zinn, J., Schumacher, J., Rosenkranz, M., Muller, D., Santorelli, S.F., et al. (2003). Op cit.

5 Kabat-Zinn, J. (1990). *Full Catastrophe Living: Using the Wisdom of your Body and Mind to Face Stress, Pain and Illness.* New York: Delacorte Press

6 Reibel, D.K., Greeson,J.M., Brainard, G.C., et al (2001). Mindfulness-based stress reduction and health-related quality of life in a heterogeneous patient population. *General Hospital Psychiatry,* 23, 183-192

7 Segal, Z., Teasdale, J., Williams, M. (2002). *Mindfulness-Based Cognitive Therapy for Depression.* New York: Guilford Press

8 Williams, Teasdale, Segal & Kabat-Zinn. Op cit.

9 Fredrickson, B., Cohn, M., Coffey, K. A, Pek, J., & Finkel, S. M. (2008). Open hearts build lives: Positive emotions induced through loving-kindness meditation, build consequential personal resources. *Journal of Personality and Social Psychology,* 95 (5), 1045–1062

10 The Buddhist Education and Information Network has guidance on loving-kindness and other meditations at www.buddhanet.net

Chapter 7

1 Carver, C.S., Scheier, M.F. and Segerstrom, S.C. (2010). Optimism. *Clinical Psychology Review.* 879–889

2 Seligman, M.E.P. (1990). *Learned Optimism.* New York: Knopf

3 Boniwell, I. (2006). *Positive Psychology in a Nutshell.* London: PWBC.

4 Norem, J.K. (2001). *The Positive Power of Negative Thinking.* New York: Basic Books.

5 Seligman. op cit.

6 Frisch, M.B. (2006). *Quality of Life Therapy.* New Jersey: John Wiley and Sons

7 Littman-Ovadia, H., and Nir, D. (2014). Looking forward

to tomorrow: The buffering effect of a daily optimism intervention. *The Journal of Positive Psychology, 9*, 122–136.

8 King, L.A. (2001). The health benefits of writing about life goals. *Personality and Social Psychology Bulletin, 27*, 798–807.

9 Sheldon, K. M., and Lyubomirsky, S. (2006). How to increase and sustain positive emotion: The effects of express expressing gratitude and visualizing best possible selves, *The Journal of Positive Psychology. 1(2)*, 73–82.

10 Schneider, S.L. (2001). In search of realistic optimism. *American Psychologist, 56(3)*, 250–263.

11 Segerstrom, S.C. (2006). *Breaking Murphy's Law.* New York: Guilford

Chapter 8

1 This description of resilience comes from Dr Chris Johnstone in *Find Your Power,* 2010, Permanent Publications

2 Masten, A.S. (2001). Ordinary magic: Resilience processes in development. *American Psychologist, 56*, 227–38

3 Reivich, K and Shatté, A. (2002). *The Resilience Factor.* New York: Broadway Books

4 Carr, A. (2004). *Positive Psychology.* Hove: Brunner-Routledge

5 Based on Zeidner, M. and Endler, N. S. (eds.) (1996). *Handbook of Coping: Theory, Research, Applications.* New York: John Wiley

6 https://ppc.sas.upenn.edu/ research/resilience-children

7 Both *The Optimistic Child* by Martin Seligman et al and *The Resilience Factor* by Karen Reivich and Andrew Shatté explore the ABC Model in detail.

8 Reivich, K. and Shatté, A. (2002). *The Resilience Factor.* New York: Broadway Books

9 Based on Burns, D.D. (1980). *Feeling Good: The New Mood Therapy* (preface by Aaron T. Beck). New York, William Morrow and Co

10 Tugade, M. and Fredrickson, B.L. (2004). Resilient individuals use positive emotions to bounce back from negative emotional experiences. *Journal of Personality and Social Psychology, 86* (2), 320–33

11 Fredrickson, B.L. (2009). *Positivity.* New York: Crown Publishers

12 Tedeschi, R.G., and Calhoun, L.G. (2004). A clinical approach to post-traumatic growth. In P.A. Linley and S. Joseph (eds.), *Positive Psychology in Practice* (pp.405–19). Hoboken, N.J.: John Wiley and Sons

13 Based on Nolen-Hoeksema, S. and Davis, C.G. (2005). Positive Responses to Loss. In C.R. Snyder and S.J. Lopez (eds). *The Handbook of Positive Psychology.* New York: Oxford University Press

14 Joseph, S (2012) *What Doesn't Kill Us.* London: Piatkus

15 Niederhoffer, K.G. and Pennebaker, J.W. (2005). Sharing one's story. In C.R. Snyder and S.J. Lopez (eds). *The Handbook of Positive Psychology.* New York: Oxford University Press

16 Pennebaker, J.W. (1989). Confession, inhibition and disease. In L. Berkowitz (ed.), *Advances in experimental social psychology, 22*, 211–44. New York:Academic Press

Chapter 9

1 Chris Peterson, author of *A Primer in Positive Psychology* (2006, NY: Oxford University Press), says that positive psychology can be summed up in three words – 'other people matter'.

2 Diener, E., and Seligman, M.E.P. (2002). Very happy people. *Psychological Science, 13*, 81–84

3 Seligman, M.E.P (1995). *The Optimistic Child*. New York: Houghton Mifflin

4 Frederickson, B. (2013). *Love 2.0*. New York: Hudson Street Press

5 Gottman, J.M. and Silver, N. (1999). *The Seven Principles for Making Marriage Work*. New York, Crown Publishers

6 Gable, S.L., Reis, H.T., Impett, E., and Asher, E.R. (2004). What do you do when things go right? The intrapersonal and interpersonal benefits of sharing positive events. *Journal of Personality and Social Psychology, 87*, 228–45

7 Ibid.

8 Goleman, D. (2006). *Social Intelligence: The New Science of Human Relationships*. New York: Bantam Books

9 Kathryn Britton's ideas on social contagion are at: positivepsychologynews.com/news/kathryn-britton/20080407704

10 Dutton, J. (2003). *Energize Your Workplace: How to Create and Sustain High-Quality Connections at Work*. San Francisco, CA: Jossey-Bass

11 Festinger, L. (1954). A theory of social comparison processes. *Human Relations, 7* (2) 117–140

12 Fredrickson, B. (2009). *Positivity: Groundbreaking Research Reveals How to Embrace the Hidden Strength of Positive Emotions, Overcome Negativity, and Thrive*. New York: Crown

13 Bryant, F.B. and Veroff, J. (2007). *Savoring: A new model of positive experiences*. Mahwah, N.J., Lawrence Erlbaum Associates, Inc.

14 Lyubomirsky, S. (2007). *The How of Happiness*. London: Sphere Books

15 Weinstein, N. and Ryan, R. (2010). When helping helps: Autonomous motivation for pro-social behaviour and its influence on well-being for the helper and recipient. *Journal of Personality and Social Psychology, 98* (2), 222–44

16 Here are some resources to get you started on spreading kindness:
www.randomactsofkindness.org
www.thekindnessoffensive.com
www.payitforwardfoundation.org

17 McCullough, M.E and van Oyen Witvliet, C. (2005). The Psychology of Forgiveness. In C.R. Snyder and S.J. Lopez (eds) *The Handbook of Positive Psychology*. New York: Oxford University Press

18 Read inspiring stories of forgiveness at www.theforgivenessproject.com

19 I can recommend *The Facebook Manager* (Management Books, 2009) by Bridget Grenville-Cleave and Jonathan Passmore on the psychology and practice of social networking

20 Dunbar, R. (2010) *How Many Friends Does One Person Need? Dunbar's Number and Other Evolutionary Quirks*. London: Faber

21 Granovetter, M. (1983). The strength of weak ties: A network theory revisited. *Sociological Theory*, 201–33

22 Canine Charter for Human Health (2008). Retrieved from www.dogstrust.org.uk

23 Nagasawa, M. et al. (2009). Dog's Gaze at Its Owner Increases Owner's Urinary Oxytocin During Social Interaction. *Hormones and Behaviour*, 55 (3), 434–41

Chapter 10

1 Korb, A. (2015). *The Upward Spiral*. Oakland: New Harbinger Publications, Inc.

2 Babyak M. Blumenthal J.A., Herman S. Khatri P., Doraiswamy M., Moore K., Craighead W.E., Baldewicz T. T., Krishnan K.R. (2000). Exercise treatment for major depression: maintenance of therapeutic benefit at 10 months. *Psychosom Med.* 62: 633–8

3 Barton J. and Pretty J. (2010). What is the best dose of nature and green exercise for mental health? A meta-study analysis. *Environmental Sci and Tech*, 44 (10), pp.3947–955

4 Loehr, J. and Schwartz, T. (2003). *The Power of Full Engagement: Managing Energy, Not Time, Is the Key to High Performance and Personal Renewal*. New York: Free Press

Chapter 11

1 Linley, A. (2008). *Average to A+*. Coventry: CAPP Press

2 Clifton, D.O. and Anderson, E.C. (2002). *Strengthsquest*. Washington: The Gallup Organisation and Peterson,

Christopher; Seligman, Martin E.P. (2004). *Character Strengths and Virtues: A handbook and classification*. Oxford: Oxford University Press

3 Seligman, M.E.P., Steen, T.A., Park, N. and Peterson, C. (2005). Positive Psychology Progress: Empirical validation of interventions. *American Psychologist*, 60, 410–21

4 Linley, A., Willars, J., Biswas-Diener, R. (2010). *The Strengths Book*. Coventry: CAPP Press

5 Peterson, Christopher; Seligman, Martin E.P. (2004). *Character strengths and virtues: A handbook and classification*. Oxford: Oxford University Press

6 Peterson, C., Park, N., and Seligman, M.E.P. (2006). Greater strengths of character and recovery from illness. *The Journal of Positive Psychology*, 1, 17–26

7 Strengths tests include the VIA (Values in Action Classification of Character Strengths; Peterson and Seligman, 2004) available at www.viacharacter.org; Realise 2 Personality Strengths Project (CAPP, 2010) can be accessed at www.strengths2020.com and Gallup's StrengthsFinder (Hodges and Clifton, 2004) is available via Gallup books and www.strengthsfinder.com

8 Seligman, M.E.P., Rashid, T., Parks, A.C. (2006). Positive Psychotherapy. *American Psychologist*, 61: 744–88.

9 Rath, T. (2007). *Strengthsfinder 2.0*. New York: The Gallup Organization

10 Read about Christine
Duvivier's inspiring work
– Appreciating Beauty in
the Bottom 80 – at
www.christineduvivier.com

Chapter 12

1 Hicks, J.A, and King, L.A.
(2009). Meaning in life as
a subjective judgment and
lived experience. *Social and
Personality Psychology Compass,
3,* 638–53

2 Frankl, V.E. (1963). *Man's Search
for Meaning.* New York: Simon
& Schuster

3 Seligman, M.E.P. (2002).
Authentic Happiness. New York:
Free Press

4 Kashdan, T.B., and McKnight,
P. E. (2009). Origins of
purpose in life: Refining our
understanding of a life well
lived. *Psychological Topics,* 18(2),
303–16

5 This exercise is based on
one from Neuro-Linguistic
Programming

6 Peterson, C., (2006). *A Primer in
Positive Psychology.* New York:
Oxford University Press

7 I first came across a version
of this activity through Neil
Crofts, author of *Authentic,
How to Make a Living by Being
Yourself.* Capstone Press

8 The U-bend of life. Why,
beyond middle age, people
get happier as they get older.
The Economist, Dec 16th 2010

9 Snyder, C.R., Rand, K.L. and
Sigmon, D.R. (2005). Hope
Theory. In Snyder, C.R., and
Lopez, S.J. (eds). *Handbook of
Positive Psychology.* London:
Oxford University Press

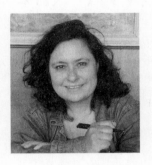

About the Author

Miriam Akhtar, MAPP, is one of the UK's leading positive psychology practitioners and authors, and was one of a hundred global experts invited to contribute to *The World Book of Happiness*. She is the author of four previous books, including *What is Post-Traumatic Growth?* for Watkins. Miriam designs and delivers well-being programmes for personal and professional development. She is also a coach, consultant, keynote speaker and visiting lecturer at a number of universities on MAPP (MSc Applied Positive Psychology) programmes.

For more information, visit:
wwww.positivepsychologytraining.co.uk

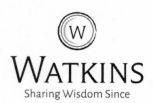

WATKINS

Sharing Wisdom Since
1893

The story of Watkins began in 1893, when scholar of esotericism John Watkins founded our bookshop, inspired by the lament of his friend and teacher Madame Blavatsky that there was nowhere in London to buy books on mysticism, occultism or metaphysics. That moment marked the birth of Watkins, soon to become the publisher of many of the leading lights of spiritual literature, including Carl Jung, Rudolf Steiner, Alice Bailey and Chögyam Trungpa.

Today, the passion at Watkins Publishing for vigorous questioning is still resolute. Our stimulating and groundbreaking list ranges from ancient traditions and complementary medicine to the latest ideas about personal development, holistic wellbeing and consciousness exploration. We remain at the cutting edge, committed to publishing books that change lives.

DISCOVER MORE AT:

www.watkinspublishing.com

Read our blog

Watch and listen to
our authors in action

Sign up to
our mailing list

We celebrate conscious, passionate, wise and happy living.
Be part of that community by visiting

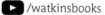 /watkinspublishing   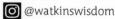 @watkinswisdom

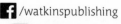 /watkinsbooks   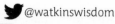 @watkinswisdom